Acknowledgements

KV-578-910

First, to my mother who provided the essential 'model of good practice' in homemaking.

Secondly, to the many kind friends who invited me into their homes and shared their experiences, hopes and fears with me.

Thirdly, to the many eminent professionals who gave most generously of their time and made available reports and records, to whom I apologise in advance for sins of omission and commission in my own reporting.

Finally, thanks are due to the following photographers whose work is shown in the picture supplement:

Michael Dowty
Bob Jones
Jeffrey Smorley
Nick Hedges
Alex Sowerby
Edward Shennan
Staff photographers at St. Lawrence's Hospital
and Pengwern Hall.

Bill Taylor

D1681107

A HOME OF THEIR OWN

HUMAN HORIZONS SERIES

A HOME
OF THEIR OWN

Victoria Shennan

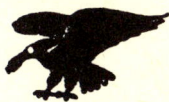

A CONDOR BOOK
SOUVENIR PRESS (E&A) LTD

Copyright © 1983 Victoria Shennan

First published 1983 by Souvenir Press (Educational & Academic) Ltd,
43 Great Russell Street, London WC1B 3PA
and simultaneously in Canada

All Rights Reserved. No part of this publication
may be reproduced, stored in a retrieval system,
or transmitted, in any form or by any means, electronic,
mechanical, photocopying, recording or otherwise without
the prior permission of the Copyright owner

ISBN 0 285 64948 5 casebound
ISBN 0 285 64949 3 paperback

Printed in Great Britain by
Ebenezer Baylis & Son Limited
The Trinity Press, Worcester, and London

Contents

Introduction

It has become fashionable to speak of mentally handicapped people as 'people just like us'. The recognition that they are people is indeed an acknowledgement of their right to consideration as citizens, with rights equal to those of others, but to insist that they are 'just like us' denies them the additional support and help which their disability demands. In common with other disabled people, mentally handicapped people cannot be expected to share fully the burdens of responsibility for others, but with preparation and training to develop their abilities, they can often be independent, responsible for themselves, and contributing members of society.

The degree of any handicap will vary from one person to another, and will be modified or aggravated by individual personalities; these same individual qualities will require many different types of provision to ensure that each handicapped person achieves some contentment and satisfaction in life.

No less than the rest of us, mentally handicapped people want to have a place of their own, where they can feel secure, where they can have their own personal possessions and be free to come and go as they wish. Some may prefer to share a house with others, some may be happiest alone, but all need the support and comfort of an accepting neighbourhood. With the increasing provision of homes for mentally handicapped people in the community the principle is no longer in question, but the definition of a home, as we understand it, is still a matter of debate.

Considerable difficulty arises in establishing an accurate assessment of the number of mentally handicapped citizens at any one time. Different criteria are involved in their classification, and although the official sources of reference are published regularly, the figures will always be fallible because of the lapse of time between collection and publication. Whereas the total population of the United Kingdom in 1980 has been calculated at 55·9 million (Government Statistical Service, 1981), the incidence of mental handicap within that figure is less easy to define; diagnosis may be made at different times in each individual's career: in infancy, at school entry, or later in life as a result of accident.

Figures quoted vary from one in a hundred babies born with some degree of handicap (which may be so mild as to cause no problems whatever), to a generally accepted figure of between three and four per thousand people who have an intelligence quotient of under 50 and are severely mentally handicapped. Obviously the assessment of the intelligence quotient implies that the person concerned has come to the attention of the relevant statutory authority, and for this reason, if accurate figures are needed, the most reliable are those for children diagnosed as in need of special education by virtue of mental handicap. Up to date statistics giving the number of children in special education, both mildly and severely handicapped, between the ages of two and nineteen years, can be obtained from the Department of Education and Science.

In this book, however, my concern is with adults, and their need for a home of their own. Many are living at home with their families and may not appear on any register. In November 1981 those living in hospitals for the mentally handicapped were stated to number 44,444 – a reduction from the figure of 52,100 quoted in 1971. At that time, 4,850 places were provided in units described as 'community residential places', and it has been estimated that 30,000 NHS places will be required in the future for people unable to live without support.

It will be apparent that the number of people we are considering is large, but with greatly varying abilities. An intelligence quotient of below 50 indicates severe retardation but does not measure personality, nor does it take account of the degree of ability of the individual, or his response to appropriate education. Any forward planning will therefore need flexibility and innovative imagination to fulfil the great range of need.

The purpose of this book is to explore some of the ways in

which a real home has been provided. Families today are small; few people live more than six persons to a home, and it is units of this size which I have sought out and visited. Among the many different types of accommodation provided there are some units of residence housing as many as twenty to forty people. These are hostels, not homes, and cannot really be considered as providing a 'home of their own'. Resident staff, especially when the ratio needs to be very high because of the disabilities of the handicapped people, also transform the living situation from that of an ordinary home into a mini institution.

A residence composed of ten profoundly handicapped people with ten staff to care for them is not a home with a small 'h'. On the other hand, a residence with two profoundly handicapped people and two who are less handicapped can become a real home, and a home for the lifetime of the residents.

The criteria of a home for the purpose of this book is a small residence, designed or adapted for the needs of the occupants, in which they have freedom and independence. Its situation should be no different from that of others, in urban or rural surroundings; there should be access to shops and public transport and the opportunity to share local amenities for education and leisure with neighbours.

The welfare benefits available to the rest of the population should take care of special needs, and the normal risks and hazards of life must be expected to afflict this group of people to the same degree as the rest of us. With proper provision, mentally handicapped people can live among us and contribute to society in a positive way. The few who truly need intensive medical care and constant supervision present an entirely separate problem, comparable only to the needs of critical illness of long duration. There is a wealth of experience already available in the management of people in this condition by the medical services.

The provision of a home of their own is not the primary concern of the hospital service, nor can it be. Comfort and constant caring must be the pattern of lives which can never achieve independence, but the very large majority of mentally handicapped people living at home today should continue to live in a home of their own for the rest of their lives, and proper planning and provision should be accepted as a duty which society owes to this special group of citizens.

PART ONE

Preparing Hospital Residents for Community
Living

1 Historical Factors

There are approximately 40,000 mentally handicapped people resident in hospitals in the United Kingdom, many of whom have spent most of their lives inside this closed world. How did this situation arise? Why is this model of care, designed so long ago, perpetuated today when, for at least fifty per cent of those still resident, it is now understood to be totally inappropriate?

Few of our present mental handicap hospitals are less than one hundred years old and most were built as a result of the Industrial Revolution of the nineteenth century. At that time there was an enormous shift of population from the rural environment into urban conurbations, when people arrived to work on the railways and in the large factories, bringing with them their entire families and among them people with physical disabilities or mental handicap. In the less stressful environment of the countryside these individuals had managed to function without too much difficulty, to at least some degree.

They were immediately a problem. The small homes which the railway owners and industrialists had built to house the workers provided minimum accommodation and were certainly not designed to provide gardens, or easy access to the rural surroundings in which mentally handicapped people had previously been able to roam with relative safety; now, in the tough working environment, they became an embarrassment. The solution was to acquire land far away from the centres of industry and to build very large institutions because, by collecting together all the requirements of care needed, the cost of provision would be reduced. They were remote from the urban centres because the land there was cheaper and not required for industrial purposes.

To these large institutions, then, were admitted all the people who were unable to contribute to the thrust of the industrial revolution. No doubt, to begin with, there was considerable distress as families were broken up in this way; but as the parents and other more able-bodied members of the family became absorbed into the industrial machine, their increasing preoccupation with the process of adjustment from a rural community to the urban environment, combined with the difficulties of travel, resulted in visits to the handicapped becoming less and less frequent. Forcibly, those who cared for them – and many were compassionate and caring people – took on the role of parents, making decisions and acting exactly as if they were in loco parentis, whether the inhabitants of the large subnormality hospitals had in fact been committed to their care or were there on an informal basis.

The first Mental Deficiency Act of 1913 attempted to regularise the position by formalising the powers of guardians of the mentally handicapped who appeared to be in need of such care. Over the years a very large number of people were accommodated in these hospitals and it became accepted that they would never go out. The pattern of their lives was dictated by the daily routine of the institution and only as changes began to appear were these modified. The surrounding land was often good farm land, and it was therefore farmed by the residents who produced their own food. There was no bar to the employment of such people within the needs of the institution and they undertook the duties needed in the laundry, kitchens and wards; in fact, the whole colony, as it was often called, was a self-supporting unit.

Enough of the old Poor Law mentality remained for it to be considered a function of the administration that they should require as little financial support as possible, and thus all the activities of the institutions were geared to self-sufficiency. In her careful study of one establishment, *Fifty Years of Harperbury Hospital*, Dr. Eileen Baranyay recounts the stages involved in setting up a hospital in the 1920s and gives a very vivid account of the conditions as they were then. She also describes the modification over the years in ideas about the management of people in subnormality units, until they came to allow for the re-integration into community life of those with the necessary ability.

It is obvious that the treatment of the less able in any community reflects the social attitudes of the general public; it is only now, with the increased knowledge of mental handicap and the growing understanding of the abilities of those with various degrees of retardation, that any movement towards community living for the majority of them has been undertaken by those outside. Provision specifically planned for them, as for other groups of people who need special attention, is still a new concept.

The staffs of the old subnormality hospitals were predominantly medical, since it was thought that mental handicap was a condition which required medical care; it was understood from the beginning, however, that it was a chronic condition and would therefore never be cured. The idea of education and special training of mentally handicapped people, to enable them to function to their full potential, was subordinate to the utilisation of their special skills within the subnormality hospital. If they were able to garden, for example, and were physically fit, they were speedily taught the practicalities of this work and became very proficient in it. Many of the old hospital farms fifty years ago produced sufficient food and of sufficient quality to feed the entire institution.

It is important to remember that, just as the Victorian households of the well-to-do employed many servants to cater for the needs of the occupants, so the same philosophy applied in the large Victorian subnormality hospitals. There were no labour-saving devices for the staff, central heating had not yet arrived and the buildings were not designed to be run by a few people. They required an enormous army of domestic staff, cooks and maintenance men, gardeners, and, to begin with, grooms and people to care for the horse-drawn means of transport. So that the idea of full occupation of everyone – what is so often described as the 'puritan work ethic' – also applied to the patients. Only the very severely mentally handicapped remained inside the wards all the time; the rest of the inmates, together with the staff, were fully employed from morning to night. There were workshops attached to every hospital, where clothing and foot-wear were made for the residents.

These hospitals were built many years ago, and to serve an age very different from our own. They remain with us today, relics of a past age, almost impossible to adapt to present day concepts, the dinosaurs of community care. Impossibly expensive to maintain, the buildings require large numbers of employees to repair and clean, and to run the out-dated kitchen and laundry facilities. Their remote situation causes transport problems, and they are staffed, in the main, by people who are totally dedicated to the care of those who must live out their days in unsuitable conditions.

It is true that children are no longer being admitted to these hospitals for life-time care, but this also means that the residents and staff are denied the compensation of the mixing of the generations enjoyed by the rest of us. New admissions to the hospital come from families who can no longer cope with lively adolescents, or from homes where the parents have died and left a bewildered mentally handicapped son or daughter, sometimes aged fifty years or more, who has never experienced life outside his or her family home.

It is a bleak prospect for the staff of the mental handicap hospitals. They are left with a population, increasingly aged and increasingly infirm, augmented by bewildered new admissions of disturbed young adults and grief-stricken older people who are admitted for no other reason than that there is nowhere else for them to go.

In spite of the White Paper *Better Services for the Mentally Handicapped*, published in 1971, which recommended that men-tally handicapped people should not be placed into hospital care if they were not in need of medical service, there are still people living in mental handicap hospitals in England today. It is estimated that over 30,000 of these are unlikely to find homes in the community in their lifetime.

Even if we accept that these people will remain in institutional care, it does not mean that they are the last to be doomed to live their whole lives in these conditions. Mentally handicapped babies are born each year, children now attending school are living with their parents, and those parents are constantly anxious about the future of their offspring when they themselves can no longer provide a home for them.

As the parents grow older they are less able to give the physical care needed by some more severely handicapped children, or to provide the constant supervision which some mentally handicapped people need. Brothers and sisters, who have helped in the daily management of the handicapped child, marry and leave home. Without the prospect of independent living for the mentally handicapped child, the parents are faced with a bleak future. To many, the only final solution still appears to be admission to a mental handicap hospital.

2 The Situation Today

The National Health Service today is faced with the problem of providing appropriate care for adult mentally handicapped people of very varying ability, some of whom have additional physical handicaps, hampered by the additional difficulties of administering huge and unsuitable buildings.

The consultative document *Care in the Community*, published by the Department of Health and Social Security, is concerned with the transfer to the community of resources at present devoted to hospital care and makes several suggestions as to how this may be done. It observes that 'there is no lack of interest in finding ways round existing problems, but other pressures on personal social services resources, and obstacles, legal and otherwise, are holding up progress'. Five ideas are proposed which give some indication of the problems experienced:

a. The health authorities selling hospital sites and donating the proceeds to the local authority for the development of smaller, residential facilities near patients' homes;

b. the development of a 'single service partnership' for services for the mentally handicapped and the pooling of health and local authority funds to finance it;

c. the conversion of local authority premises into hostels to accommodate people inappropriately cared for in hospital, with the local authority staffing and running the hostel and the health authority meeting the cost on a contractual basis and being responsible for selecting the people to be transferred;

d. the sale of a NHS tuberculosis hostel to a housing association, the health authority continuing to pay for people using the hostel;

e. converting hospital 'villas' to hostels which the residents rent from the health authority, using their supplementary benefits to pay for food and accommodation.

One aspect which is comparatively new is that disabled people of all degrees of handicap are now in receipt of personal incomes from state benefits. Whilst resident in hospital these payments are suspended, since the general principle is that no individual can receive a double benefit. If he is provided with living accommodation, food, heating and other essential services, the state benefit which would cover these needs if he were living in the community is withdrawn. The fact that mentally handicapped people qualify for non-contributory invalid pensions, mobility allowances and, in some cases, attendance allowance, has made it financially possible to consider alternative means of residence for small groups who, by pooling their resources of money and ability, can become a self-supporting household.

The idea that mentally handicapped people should live as our neighbours in ordinary houses is still a revolutionary concept. The barriers of fear and prejudice still produce opposition to local schemes in many areas. Provision for other groups of people with special housing needs – elderly people, orphaned children, physically handicapped people – has for many years been accepted by local authorities. Few areas do not now have some allocation of old people's bungalows, flats or residential homes, and most have provided a children's home in their new housing estates.

The idea that in order to be economically viable a 'Home' must be a large building, with several staff members, purpose-built for residents with special needs, began to be challenged during the last two decades. Existing 'Homes' were reorganised on a family group basis, creating an artificial family of six to eight children of varying ages, with houseparents of both sexes, replacing the old rigid pattern of caring for twenty or more infants in nurseries, moving them to a children's unit at school age and, as they left school, transferring them again into a different residential unit. Elderly people were gradually accommodated in small, individual flats under the supervision of wardens, as an alternative to the 'Old People's Homes'.

In the years which led up to present-day community housing, mentally handicapped people had little special provision designed especially for their needs; their condition is not notifiable, in statutory terms. If they were in the categories laid down under the various modifications and amendments of the Mental Deficiency Act of 1913, and the revisions of that Act embodied in the Mental Health Act of 1959, then the local authority was required to provide for the equipment and maintenance of residential accommodation for them, and staff for their care.

Prior to the NHS re-organisation of 1974 the identification of those in need of such accommodation and care was carried out by mental health welfare officers, and since there was no statutory duty to identify and register people as mentally handicapped, many children and adults continued to live at home, receiving only family care and some education and training at Junior Training Centres set up by the local authority health service.

The obligation to provide residential accommodation was often interpreted as directing the child or adult whose needs could not be met at home into the nearest subnormality hospital. Some authorities did attempt to provide hostel-type accommodation for mentally handicapped people; as stated in the Introduction, at the time of publication of the White Paper *Better Services for the Mentally Handicapped* in 1971, the number of places provided, nationwide, in all types of community care residence, was given as 4,850, as opposed to 52,100 places in mental handicap hospitals.

No estimate of the numbers of people currently living at home with families was possible, because of the fears of parents of the stigma still attached to all forms of mental handicap and illness – the two conditions being confused in the minds of most people. Many families cared for mentally handicapped family members of all ages under conditions of secrecy and virtual isolation, and carried this burden, without help, until circumstances made it impossible to continue.

Today, with only limited accommodation provided by local authorities, the alternatives for parents remain few, and in most cases, only two. Private or voluntary organisations provide a range of residences, from guest houses and nursing homes to village communities. Payment for these services varies from acceptance of the full cost by the family, or with assistance provided by various charitable trusts, and in some cases, modest amounts from the local authority concerned. The hospital, on the other hand, accepts full responsibility for the resident and he or she ceases to be a financial charge either to the family or to the local authority.

Some areas do not have a mental handicap hospital in their home area, and admissions are made into hospitals at a considerable distance. Family links can only be maintained with great difficulty, and home visits for short break periods often cease after childhood. Separation from the family and the neighbourhood from which the mentally handicapped person originally came is the rule rather than the exception for older residents in mental handicap hospitals, unless the family lives reasonably near. The very isolation of so many large hospitals is aggravated today by the reduction of public transport systems.

After struggling to maintain contact with children in hospital for many years, parents become too old to undertake the journeys and the links with family, friends and neighbours are finally severed. Those several thousands of people who have been in hospital residences for over thirty years will remain there; they are the lost generations.

Our task is to ensure that we do not perpetuate past errors by failing to look far enough ahead when we plan today for tomorrow.

3　One Man's Story

The inspiration for this book was provided by my friend, Joseph Deacon. I first met him in 1973, when he was 53 years old, and we remained in close contact until his death in December 1981. During those few years I visited him frequently, at first in the ward of a mental handicap hospital in which he had spent many years of his life.

The building was typical of its kind – huge and impersonal, with long wards and endless corridors, out of date equipment and a population of hundreds of men and women, all affected with mental handicap in varying degrees of severity. Some, like Joseph Deacon, were so severely and doubly handicapped with both mental and physical disabilities that, without someone to give total care, they would undoubtedly have died in childhood. These profoundly afflicted men and women spent most of their time in beds and wheelchairs, only able to savour the pleasure of the gardens if their nurses or friends wheeled them outside the long wards or established them on the balconies. Many could not feed themselves, or perform the simplest bodily functions without help.

Their daily lives were dependent upon the quality of the staff around them, and many of the men I met as friends of Joey (as everyone came to call him) regarded certain members of the nursing staff almost as the parents they had, in some cases, never known, turning to them for advice and comfort in distress.

The staff of St. Lawrence's Hospital, where Joey and his friends lived out their lives, were engaged in a continuous and wearing struggle to adapt the archaic hospital and its outmoded system to contemporary living, and to improve the lives of those who had no other home. Some of the residents would always be so physically afflicted that, without the total and dedicated commitment of others, life, even in a specially built house, would not be possible.

On the face of it, Joseph Deacon would most certainly have been placed in this category. Yet I was privileged to see him removed from the ward which had for so long been his home and installed in a bungalow of his own, cared for by his friends, where he could spend the last years of his life living as he had always dreamt of being able to do.

Observing the fulfilment of what had seemed an impossible dream introduced me to the whole field of residence outside hospitals for mentally handicapped people. For this experience I am deeply indebted to Joey and his friends, and especially to Dr. Geoffrey Harris who finally achieved his aim of proving that independent living was possible, given full commitment and support. His unswerving determination enabled him to surmount all obstacles in pursuit of his goal.

The small group of bungalows standing within the grounds of the old hospital are not far away in terms of physical distance, but the life style of the residents in these bungalows is as far removed from that of the wards from which they have come as if they had been transported from another planet.

I had been working in the field of mental handicap for many years, without much daily contact with mentally handicapped people themselves, when I was given the privilege of producing Joseph Deacon's book. He had been a patient in a subnormality hospital for over fifty years, and my friendship with him enabled me to understand, in some small way, exactly what mental handicap really means to those afflicted in this way. Joey was totally without speech and quadruply spastic, quite unable to perform any of the simplest functions of living for himself. He had three friends, and the family of four men between them managed to produce the book, *Tongue Tied*. It is still being printed all over the world, in several languages, and the film, which was made from the book by the BBC 'Horizon' team, won an international award and made friends for Joey wherever it was shown. This film alone contributed a great deal to the change in public opinion about mentally handicapped people in every country in which it was shown.

I worked very closely with the author during the time the book was being produced and on several occasions visited the sub-normality hospital in which he lived, in order to clarify points and do the kind of work that an editor does with any other author. I achieved a very warm relationship with the little group of friends and found myself in particular sympathy with Joseph Deacon. We were both writers and were close to each other in age, so we shared many memories of past experiences. Joey was of normal intelligence but his three friends were each severely mentally handicapped.

At the Press reception to launch his book, a reporter asked Joey, through his interpreter, Ernie, what would he have liked to do had he not been born handicapped. His answer was immediate: 'I would have liked to travel, to see much more of the world.' When asked if he had any other ambitions in life, he responded equally promptly: 'To live in a home of my own.' I think it was at that moment that I, at least, completely understood that mentally handicapped and other disabled people *are* indeed people like us. They share the universal, fundamental desire for a home of one's own, a private place, a place to which we can retreat, where we can be ourselves, which will give us protection and shelter not only from the climate and environment but from the many stresses and strains of life; a place where we can renew ourselves, where we can be truly ourselves.

Certainly, in the crowded reception room at the Waldorf Hotel, with the representatives of the Press and the media around us, as Joey talked about his hopes of living one day in a home of his own, he expressed an emotion which is familiar to every one of us and unites us in our common humanity.

He had spent fifty years of his life in a large institution, and when I first met him I was able to see how he and his friends had created a tiny module of a home of their own, in a corner of an outside verandah which the hospital had placed at the disposal of the four men. Here they had their own small personal possessions: a budgerigar in a cage, some posters, letters and postcards that had been sent to them. After the publication of the book, this corner became embellished with an extraordinary number of items from all over the world, including a framed letter from Her Majesty the Queen.

The story of how Joey's home of his own came about is unique, but the stages and steps and the problems which were encountered as it came into being will be experienced by many other people who are mentally handicapped, and probably by many physically handicapped people as well; all those who have always been thought of as only able to support life in an institution, with all the resources of medical care around them and a large staff to give them the day-to-day attention that they need. Joey's story proves that it is not only *possible* for a man who is totally unable to care for himself to live in his own home, but that it is possible to do so by using untrained people who have been taught the necessary skills to look after their friends.

If further proof were needed that Joey and his friends were, indeed, people like us, the very first obstacle to be surmounted in providing them with a home of their own was money. They themselves had only the small allowance which is made by law to people who are permanently resident in a hospital. The book at that time was unpublished, and unsold, and there was no guarantee of any income from it.

As most authors will know, income from writing is problematic, to say the least. It could not, at that time, have been thought that Joey's book would prove such a success or that the income from it would enable small luxuries to be added to the lives of the friends and permit them to travel as they had wished. It was unlikely that there would ever be enough money from the sale of a book of such limited appeal to provide the finance needed to purchase land to build a house; in any case, Joey's own physical condition made such a project highly unlikely.

The story of how the money arrived is a small miracle. Two years after the publication of the book, Joey was able to travel on the continent from the income which it provided. At that time travelling with such a severely handicapped man was in the nature of a pioneering experiment, and the preparations were like those for an expedition up the Amazon. Joey had to travel in his special wheelchair, as did his friend, Ernie. Their two able-bodied friends helped in the lifting and transportation but someone had to drive the bus or the conveyance – the ambulance in the first instance – which would take them to the port of departure. There had to be special arrangements to take them across the Channel, to receive them on the other side and to facilitate both their travel and their accommodation when they were in other countries. They were always accompanied by Dr. Geoffrey Harris, physician in charge of the particular department of the hospital where Joey at that time was resident.

Geoffrey Harris made all these things possible. He dealt with the necessary paperwork which would allow Joey to travel outside the hospital with his friends. He assisted in the careful administration and dosage of the drugs which made the journey tolerable and which controlled Joey's spasticity sufficiently for him to enjoy the days and a quiet sleep at the end of them.

Throughout the years that followed, their annual holiday to the place of their own choice was always arranged by Geoffrey Harris who gave up his own holiday time and accompanied the party at his own expense, in order to help Joey and his friends take a holiday like everyone else.

In 1976 they were visiting Amsterdam, and the BBC film 'Joey', based on the book, had recently been screened in Holland. As Joey and his friends sat outside in a street café they were approached by a group of people who greeted him, saying, 'Hello, Joey, we know you, we've seen you on the television.' The word soon spread and, later in the day, an outside broadcast television team of one of the Dutch stations came and recorded a short interview with Joey and his friends. This programme, of only seven to ten minutes' duration, was screened in Holland at Christmas time. It was not transmitted as an appeal and no special results from the programme were expected by the team who made it, but the response was incredible. By the next morning money was being sent to the television station for Joey Deacon and his friends, and over the next few months a sum of about £50,000 was collected. St. Lawrence's Hospital, Caterham, was asked to take charge of the money and administer it for Joey. This they were not able to do, as under the National Health Service rules they could not administer particular funds for an individual patient.

They then applied to the National – now Royal – Society for Mentally Handicapped Children and Adults (Mencap), as publishers of the book, to ask if they could administer this fund for the particular needs of Mr. Deacon. As a national charity Mencap had no machinery by which this enterprise could be handled for one individual. By the general terms of charitable status Mencap is obliged to look after *all* mentally handicapped people and their families, not to give attention to one particular person. So the first dilemma was how this finance could be managed and how it could be dispensed. Fortunately, at St. Lawrence's, there existed an organisation of Friends of the Hospital who accepted the responsibility of holding funds, and it was decided that the money should be used to build the first of a series of experimental living units which the Hospital had thought for some time should be provided for patients who, it was considered, need not be housed inside the wards of a hospital.

The first big obstacle, of course, was the land. Where was this house to be sited? To buy a plot in the community was impracticable for a number of reasons. A special bungalow or house had to be designed, since one of the intended residents was totally disabled and another very severely disabled. There was the difficulty of obtaining planning permission, and at that time the authorities concerned were very well aware of the opposition they would encounter from the neighbourhood if it were suggested that a specially built house should be set down in the centre of an ordinary housing estate to house people from the subnormality hospital. No one at that time could conceive that people who had been in hospital for fifty years were 'people like us'.

The hospital, like many other large subnormality hospitals of the time, had a great deal of land around it; some of it had in the past been farmed and now lay idle. There was even a large stretch immediately adjoining a public road, eminently suitable for building houses. It was, of course, land in the ownership of the National Health Service, and at that time it was not considered practicable that it should be sold off or used for any purpose other than for that which it was designed. But nevertheless, with some considerable difficulty, permission was at last obtained to build a collection of bungalows, one of which would be for Joey and his friends and the others for other patients who, it was felt, could live in small units with a little support.

The situation at St. Lawrence's Hospital was common to all such institutions: a diminishing number of profoundly handicapped people, many very elderly, housed in large premises almost impossible to staff and maintain, with new admissions arriving on the death of elderly parents who had cared for their mentally handicapped children at home. These new arrivals were, in many cases, capable of living in ordinary homes in the community, with a little help, but because suitable accommodation was not being provided the hospital still remained as the final desperate resource.

Dr. Geoffrey Harris explained to me in a long interview how the first bungalows were built and the many obstacles overcome. Since his was the driving force, I cannot do better than quote him.

I went to the Area Management Team of the Authority and I said, 'Look, we have the money now, where do we go from here?' They agreed that we could build. We talked a lot about the site, and we decided together that this was the only practical one because any other area of the hospital was too far away from it to be possible to keep any kind of eye on it. In those days we felt we needed to keep an eye on the site and have it within reasonable distance. So we settled on the place and everybody agreed on that.

Then somebody said, 'Ah, but we must have planning permission,' and there was a lot of discussion about whether we really *needed* it; but in the end it was decided that it would be right to ask for permission, so we went to Tandridge Council and said, 'Please could we build twelve bungalows on this site,' and they said 'No'. To cut a long story short, that decision was backed up by the Surrey County Council; they also said 'No'.

There were three major objections which they put to us,

supported by a couple of letters from local residents, which I
saw:

1. That it would spoil the view from the road. (This road
    has a bank of trees which screen the bungalows, so that
    was rubbish.)
2. That this was going to create a lot of extra noise for
    people in Chaldon Road (although it was fenced off
    from the hospital grounds and access was denied to us).
3. That this was Green Belt and planning permission
    could not be given to build on Green Belt (in spite of
    the fact that not only was it hospital land, but there was
    building all round that field, on three sides, including
    the side facing the open country where there is a school
    and other buildings).

So we felt the whole objection was unjustified. We appealed
and they turned the appeal down; we had to go to the Ministry
of the Environment for a decision, and *they* came down and we
all sat round a table: the Health Authority, the Ministry of the
Environment and the Hospital. The Ministry of the Environment later wrote to us and said, 'Yes, you can build
twelve bungalows.'

This summary of these initial difficulties covers months of set-
backs, rebuffs and bureaucratic procedures which wasted
valuable time. Meanwhile the four friends waited impatiently for
signs of progress.

The hospital authorities had already been convinced that, if
funds were available, they could, by providing a pilot project in
independent living, prove the viability of moving the majority of
people from the institutional wards into smaller private homes.
The initial donation from the Dutch people provided the spur.
As Geoffrey Harris told me:

The fund rose to about £57,000, and having got that much
money and feeling that it was, at that time, enough for more
than one building, we then decided, 'Let's go for the three
bungalows.' We went to the King's Fund and they said, 'We'll
give you £25,000.' By that time, the Area Health Authority

had said, 'Right, that's probably enough, but we'll meet the difference'. They did not know when they said this that the difference was going to be yet another £30,000, but they met us at the end of the day.

A large part of that money went for the initial groundwork, sewers, etc., but we had a road to the site from within the grounds, though no direct access onto the public highway. I hope that one day we might have access to Chaldon Road, which is at present not permitted. Our bungalows would then be really part of the neighbourhood.

All the time the bungalows were being built, there was a steadily improving climate of public opinion towards residence outside the mental handicap hospitals. Long stay residents were being referred to the local authorities responsible for them and were being approached by social work staff who assessed their abilities and the possibility of discharging them to the hostels which some authorities had built in the years following the White Paper of 1971.

Tom and Michael, who were already able to move around and go outside the walls for shopping and entertainment, were offered this kind of accommodation – hostels providing the chance of living in the community. The four friends discussed the possibility together and informed the hospital that they did not wish to be separated. They would prefer, all four, to continue to live in St. Lawrence's Hospital which had become their home and in which they had achieved some degree of independent living.

When the suggestion of building a bungalow for Joey arose, it was obvious that it had to be considered as a bungalow for a group of four, and for the four particular people who made a family. The constitution of this small group was, in fact, ideal, although it may not have appeared to be so at first sight. There were two men who always needed wheelchairs, even for short distances, one of whom, Joey, being quadruply spastic, could do absolutely nothing for himself. His friend, Ernie, was the only person of the group who could understand the sounds which Joey made in lieu of speech. However, Tom, who had worked in a sawmill until his eighteenth birthday and had only been admitted to the hospital on the death of his parents, was physically able. His intelligence was just below 50, but he had a great deal of that uncommon gift, common sense, was able-bodied and could anticipate difficulties, particularly those concerned with simple mechanics like the gas or electric stoves and other appliances, and he could put them right if the fault was a minor one. His good mechanical sense, allied to his common sense, made him an essential member of the team.

For a long time I thought that Michael, the fourth member, was a 'passenger'. He is not robust, his intelligence is low and his speech is difficult. However, he can write a few words and can compose a letter which is intelligible to those who receive it. With patient listening he can convey his opinions and recount what has happened during the day. It was a long time before I saw how essential to the other three was the place of Michael in the team.

Michael had to be 'looked after' and the other three men looked after him admirably. On one occasion I was present when he had gone out for the evening and not returned. The three friends discussed what might have happened to him and what should be done if he did not return; their anxiety and affection for this weaker member of their team was evident. We all need someone to care for. Joey's needs were physical and he had to be cared for daily by the others in the team. Michael's needs are not physical, he can look after himself very well, wash, shave, find food and cook for himself, but he has a greater need of emotional support and care than any of the others in the group. In supplying it the needs of the others were met in their turn.

The importance of this form of selection for a happy and successful family life cannot be forgotten by those who must make the provision. The four friends had their arguments, they disagreed on many subjects, but they were quicker to come to a compromise agreement than most of us because they were willing to give way to each other and to see the practical advantages of not compromising their own personal needs. This tolerance was the result of living closely together in hospital over many years.

The physical environment of the house is equally important. If sufficient attention is not given to the details of living, extra stress and annoyance is caused. For example, when the four friends were being trained in the hospital for the routine duties of cooking, housekeeping and looking after the others, these mainly fell upon Tom. When I first saw them in their new home Tom told me, showing the stove which had been supplied, 'This electric cooker has only got two rings. I was taught on one with four, it's very difficult to cook for us all on two rings.' This seems a simple point and Tom was in no way carping or criticising what the authority had provided, but it was a silly omission. Even if it was only a temporary measure it made the preparation of their own food extraordinarily difficult. Being able to prepare one's own meals is an absolute keystone in this kind of living. To move into a small unit and have all your meals delivered to the door is *not* living like other people, nor does it provide the opportunity to make mistakes in diet and to indulge personal tastes.

One would have thought that to share a house with someone like Joey, who had great difficulty in swallowing and whose food had previously been prepared in the diet kitchens of the hospital, would have presented enormous problems. It proved perfectly simple for Joey to be fed by Tom because Tom understood perfectly the difficulties which would be presented by different foods. All the meals were cooked by Tom and he used a liquidiser for Joey's meals, and took the liquidiser with him when they went on holiday.

I remember one occasion when they were giving a party. The four men decided to entertain the nurses who had cared for them before they left the hospital. There was a bar set up and guests like myself were greeted and asked what they would like to drink. When I asked for a sherry, Tom went off and came back with a tray on which there were glasses of sherry. He produced from his pocket a feeding cup, transferred the sherry for Joey into this then went off to greet another group of friends, leaving me with the feeding cup containing Joey's sherry and my own sherry in a glass. It was with considerable trepidation that I attempted to give Joey his sherry, but I discovered quite quickly that if I trickled the sherry down the inside of his cheek and gave him time to swallow it, he got on very well. In fact, I heard the next day that in the course of the evening Joey had had several sherries and had enjoyed the party in the same spirit as the rest of the guests – which is to say, he became as merry as the rest. A small incident, but it does show that many of the skills of nursing and caring, feeding and looking after people who have special needs are not exclusively the prorogative of professionals. Sometimes an intuitive understanding of what is required can prompt ordinary members of the family to find a way of supplying it.

Although the bungalow for the four friends was specially planned for them and purpose-built for their needs, insufficient information had been given to the architect. For example, it was assumed that because of Joey's condition he would need daily nursing care. Therefore the bath was designed on the same lines as the baths in the institution. It was raised in order to spare the nurse who would be lifting the men in and out of the bath, and it was accessible on all sides. In practice, Michael and Tom, who were responsible for lifting Joey and Ernie in and out of the bath, would have found it very much simpler if they had had an ordinary low bath of the kind in use in houses, although it was better for them to be able to reach it from both sides. Taking another example, it was assumed that all their laundry would be handled by the hospital laundry and therefore no airing cupboard or washing machine were provided. The men washed their jumpers and jerseys in the kitchen sink extremely efficiently, but in order to dry them they were obliged to drape them on the radiators.

Ernie had an electric car as well as a wheelchair with rechargeable batteries, and one was also supplied for Joey. This meant that they needed garage space for the car and chairs, and they also needed a socket outlet, so that the batteries could be recharged. This had not been supplied, and in the winter of my first visit to them, I found them with the windows open so that a lead could be brought in from outside to charge up the battery.

There were other difficulties similar to those that occur even in ordinary homes that are purpose built; there are things which the planners would like to change when they see the actual living conditions. On the whole the house was comfortable for them and they themselves made no criticisms. The drawbacks I have mentioned were those I observed for myself and I asked if they felt them difficult when they obviously found them so.

They could have a meal on the wards where they used to live, at any time, if they chose, but generally they preferred to go to the stores once or twice a week and draw the basic requirements for their own meals. They were still nominally hospital residents and as such received the quantity of food which would be allocated to them on the usual scales for each patient. Tom enjoyed cooking and offering hospitality to visitors, and he also organised the other household chores.

In looking after themselves, mentally handicapped people acquire meaningful occupation and have the satisfaction of independence. Employment of some kind, as distinct from work for which they receive pay, is essential for even the most profoundly mentally handicapped people, no less than the physically disabled. A life of enforced idleness and boredom is not progress, in any sense. It can be salutary to look back on a time where everyone was toiling industriously from sun-up to sun-set, and contrast it with the impression one receives on visiting wards today. Groups of patients can still be found, sitting apathetically in front of a television set without occupation, while around them the wards show evidence of the need for small domestic duties which are not being performed, due to lack of staff. Progress takes very many different forms.

The world of the four friends continued to expand after the official opening of their home. The BBC television team, 'Blue Peter', built a fourth bungalow as the result of a national appeal, and this will house the last few remaining child patients from St. Lawrence's Hospital.

In the summer of 1979 I visited them on holiday in Blackpool. The earlier holidays in France, Switzerland and Holland had been completely successful, but the overseas journeys had necessitated some staff help, and the four friends decided to have a holiday in a U.K. resort. At the guest house in Blackpool they had help only from Geoffrey Harris and his wife. On my visit I was able to stay with the group for one evening so that Geoffrey Harris could be free. Because of the wheelchairs and consequent difficulty in premises not ideally suited for mobility, the friends were never left without some additional support, but in practice I soon found that other guests and holidaymakers were only too ready to do whatever might be needed to help.

On the evening that I was there Michael had set off for a drink at a nearby public house. Joey, Ernie, Tom and I were seated in the glassed-in conservatory facing the sea, watching the tram-cars, which carried an advertising slogan for 'Ernie', the Premium Bond selection machine. It gave us all much amusement to see passing at intervals the illuminated sign 'Ernie is here'. Our evening was further enlivened by the proprietor's dog, a huge Irish Wolfhound, which joined the party, resting his head on Joey's shoulder. We were then joined by a uniformed inspector of police who interviewed the proprietor, in our hearing, for evidence of vandalism that had been perpetrated that day in the hotel by a gang of youths.

Joey and his friends listened with growing indignation to the proprietor's excited and dramatic account of doors smashed, guests' clothes slashed and fights between rival gangs – it was a Bank Holiday weekend.

When the proprietor and the inspector left, Tom gave me his views on such behaviour and Joey, through Ernie, made it very apparent that they were aware of incidents of this kind which had been reported in the press and on television and had very decided views on the cause and treatment. They were all quite unanimous that the parents and families concerned were to blame for not teaching the perpetrators better ways. They discussed among themselves the values they had been given in the hospital – the church services and the example of the nursing staff of years gone by. 'We had to be shown right from wrong!'

As time passed and Michael did not return, they began to be concerned about him. It was not yet dark, about 9.30 p.m., and the promenade was brightly lit. They debated about going out to look for him. Tom said it would be a waste of time as he could be anywhere. They explained to me that they were anxious because he was sometimes careless about mixing his drinks or about his drinking companions. 'There are some very funny people about, you know,' they said. 'Kidnappers, even.' When I suggested that perhaps I could look in to the nearest pub to see if he was there, Tom said, 'You can't go on your own, and if I came with you we'd have to leave Ernie and Joey on their own, so we'll just have to wait.'

I treasure the memory of that evening with them, companionably discussing issues of the day as we waited for the errant Michael, who duly arrived, slightly the worse for wear, just after 10 p.m. and was hastily despatched to bed by Tom. We were all quietly partaking of the hotel's bed-time tea-tray when Geoffrey Harris returned, to be acquainted with the account of the police visit and the events of the day which we had learnt from his investigations. 'Michael's in bed, Geoff,' said Tom, and quietly, aside to me, 'No need to worry Dr. Harris about him being out.'

In the summer of 1981 they had been in residence for two years, and when I saw them then it was obvious that the bungalow had now become a real home. Living there had both changed their reactions to each other and expanded their world. They now had immediate neighbours: two other bungalows occupied by residents from the hospital, and the fourth building going up. The policy today is not to admit children to such hospitals and to remove those who have been cared for there for some time into more appropriate surroundings. The 'Blue Peter' bungalow has made this possible at St. Lawrence's.

Many of the difficulties which I had observed on earlier visits had by now been overcome. For example, there was a larger cooker and also a washing machine; although they could if they wished have their sheets and towels and personal laundry done by the hospital, they preferred to wash their ordinary clothing in the way that the rest of us do. The house had stood up very well to the two years of occupation and was in good decorative order; many of the small annoyances had been overcome. There was a garage now outside for the wheelchairs and Ernie's electric car. The draughtproofing had been improved and the bath had been lowered to make life easier for the bathing of the two handicapped men. The physical conditions under which they lived were as near ideally suited to them as it was possible to contrive. They had, for example, a large hobby room which was very necessary because here they kept the typewriter on which they still produced their original and creative writing. They had had another story published, in an American journal, about two spastics who decide to marry, and they also indulged in many other hobbies and had special pleasure in a video recorder which they used expertly.

Tom still did all the house work to a standard which many women would envy. The bedrooms of Ernie and Joey were orderly and they had their own possessions around them. What was interesting to me on this occasion was that the problem uppermost in their minds was not one concerned with their physical environment, but a problem involving Michael. Michael, as I have already described, is more independent in some ways than the others. He has always been able to come and go from the hospital as he wished and has been accustomed to going on quite long bus rides and to visiting the local pubs for a drink. He has several friends outside the hospital. Nevertheless, he was very closely involved with the other three men who provided him with the family support which he needed.

The movement to get people out of hospital and into the community was gathering momentum, and Michael, being a responsibility of one of the larger London boroughs, had been offered the chance, by that social services department, of a place much nearer the centre of the City in a hostel with other people. The four men were greatly concerned about the problem which would have to be faced if he decided to accept the place. They were scrupulously fair and several times said to Michael, 'It is your choice, Michael. We don't want to stand in your way if you want to go out.'

Michael told me that he had been asked if he wanted to go but, as he explained, he had never been in a hostel and had no idea what it was like. He appealed to Ernie. Ernie has had a greater experience of life through many friends and he was quite definite that life in a hostel was not likely to suit Michael. As he put it, 'There will be rules, you will have to do what you are told, not like here where you do what you like.' Michael sat on the edge of his bed looking very anxious and said to me that perhaps he would like to go and live in the City because it would be nearer his mother. Tom then said, 'But your mother is over 70 years old. Suppose when you get there she dies. Then you will be all on your own again and you won't have the same kind of friends as you've got here.' But they constantly reassured him that it was his choice.

When he had gone out for a walk, Tom said to me, 'I don't know how Michael will manage really, because he does need looking after. You see, when he goes out from here we all tell him to be careful who he talks to in the pub and not to have too many drinks, and we stay up till he comes back. What would happen to him in the City? If he is in a big town, no one will know where he is or what he is doing.'

Ernie brought up another point. 'If Michael moved out we would have to have another person to take his place in this bungalow, and they might not get on with us.' Tom immediately said, 'Well we mustn't be selfish. I know it would not suit us but we've got to think of what suits Michael.' It seemed that Michael had had a visitor, a young social worker from his area, who had put the alternatives to him to the best of her ability, and had offered to take Michael to visit the hostel in which he was being offered a place so that he might make a decision. It was obvious to me that there was no way that Michael could make an informed choice. He had no experience of living anywhere else except in the hospital and had received very careful preparation to move into this particular bungalow with the three men who had been part of his life for many years.

Many mentally handicapped people have great difficulty in transferring learning skills from one situation to another and, as an observer, I could see many problems which would arise. I was very impressed by the mature and unselfish way in which the other three men had tackled this problem and were doing their best to be as objective and supportive as they could be.

We discussed other situations which had arisen since they had been living together and I found that they all managed extremely well with their shopping and cooking, and that their general health appeared to be as good as it had been when they were living under much stricter medical supervision. However, they received regular visits from Dr. Harris who acted as their general practitioner and probably gave them more personal medical care than most of us receive.

They had a system whereby they could call the hospital maintenance staff either for general repairs or for emergencies such as trouble with water or their appliances; the maintenance men would arrive and deal with an emergency very quickly.

While I was there a woman from a neighbouring bungalow came in to talk and have a cup of tea with us, and explained that two of her fellow residents were undergoing hospital treatment for some minor ailments which required an anaesthetic and would be returning when the hospital felt that they were fit to do so. In the event they both returned while I was still with Joey and his friends, and the lady came back again to say that she thought they looked a bit unsteady, so she had advised them to undress and get into bed and they were now both asleep.

Even minor medical emergencies can be dealt with in this way, for the common sense of mentally handicapped people is at least as caring and functional as that of others. Perhaps it is more so, since they are more actively concerned about each other and, as we have already suggested, have an intuitive knowledge of what their friends, some of whom have no speech, require at a particular moment.

Around the area of the bungalows there was a fair amount of land due to be laid out as gardens, and this was already proceeding. Joey and his friends were delighted to hear that children were going to be in the fourth house; this mixing of the generations again is one of the features which gives a greater degree of normality to the lives of mentally handicapped people, no less than the rest of us.

We talked about expenses and the use of the various allowances to which the group were entitled. They told me that they had more than sufficient money for their needs, and that when they wanted to go to visit friends at some considerable distance, they hired a taxi from a particular driver who knew them, all four setting off to visit the relatives and friends of any one of the group; they arranged all this for themselves. They had two television sets, and when these needed repair they arranged that too and paid for it from their own money.

They had obviously achieved a life within the sheltered environment of the hospital community and were looked after extremely well by the services provided by the central hospital unit. Certainly, Joey could not exist in a bungalow in the community without recourse to a medical centre which could provide for emergency treatment. During my visit Dr. Harris called and observed that Joey had some swelling of the legs and arm; he immediately arranged for him to go for a check-up within two or three days. This kind of supervision is particularly needed for the totally afflicted patient. People with profound and severe physical defects, in addition to their mental handicap, complicated, as in Joey's case, by lack of speech, should certainly be in the care of people who are aware of any difficulty.

I asked Geoffrey Harris how the hospital had selected the residents for the other bungalows and whether they had experienced any problems. This was his reply:

Well, the first person we had, who wanted to try living off the ward, did not last very long. It was not the fault of the other members of the group because this particular person missed her old environment and her ward sister, for whom she had a deep affection; she just wanted to go back. We then tried somebody else who proved to be incompatible, was just rather difficult, and who did not get on with the others.

The third attempt was successful. The four settled down quite happily afterwards and the present group works very well. There haven't been any major difficulties – we can say that quite honestly – and this is fortunate. We have met difficulties, but they have been minor ones of the kind where we found equipment was not right or something was wrong about the bungalow, and we had to make minor alterations.

The Joey four, Joey, Tom, Michael and Ernie, had been together all the time, and worked on the book and the film. We decided when we looked for other groups of four that we wanted to make certain that we were offering housing as a priority for people who were spastic.

When the project got under way we were looking for people who could not only benefit from such housing but who could not easily have found housing anywhere else; and we felt that spastics were the kind of people who would be most difficult to house, because of their physical disabilities. There is not enough provision for physically disabled people, so both the first groups had spastics in them.

Now, we have one house with two spastic men and two mentally handicapped able-bodied women, one of whom is very capable in all ways but beyond the age where we are going to find a place for her outside the hospital. The two ladies look after the two spastic men and they have formed a very close group of four. We found two others for whom it would not be easy to find outside accommodation, namely a married couple, where neither had a very high level of intelligence – the wife probably higher than the husband – and we wanted to give them a chance to get married and have a married life. So we decided that we would try them in a bungalow, and *they* now support two other ladies who are less able.

In St. Lawrence's Hospital, at the time when Joey, and later his friends, were admitted, all residents had duties to perform. Joey recorded in his book that he worked in the hospital industrial units like everyone else, to the limit of his capacity. He worked in the mat shop from 1935, for sixteen years, and managed to select colours required for the weavers with the help of Ernie; and even several years later, in 1960, he was taken daily to the Training Centre and managed to make a table runner on a loom which was shown in a local exhibition and won a prize.

Within the limits of the knowledge available at the time, residents were given employment suited to their abilities, a simple code of behaviour and acceptance of duties. They were able to build upon this framework to achieve independent lives, working together and sharing their abilities to best advantage.

Less than a month after this visit, on 8th December 1981, Joey Deacon died. He was able to live in his home, with his friends, almost until the very end of his life. His contribution to the increased understanding of people everywhere of the plight of mentally handicapped people is impossible to measure.

His friends were understandably grief stricken at his loss. The floral tributes from all who knew him, personally or by reputation, had been placed, at his friends' request, surrounding the little bungalow and covering the winter ground. They took me round and pointed out the names of various senders with affection.

Joey had bequeathed all his possessions to Ernie, so there was no physical change inside their home. The framed translations of his book hung on the sitting room wall, the photographs and awards still embellished the hobbies room, the budgerigar chirruped in his cage.

They had invited a fourth person to share their home, a fellow resident of Ward C1, who had often helped them. 'Joey would want us to get on with it,' said Tom.

I looked back at the little group in the doorway as I left them. Joey had given a perfect example of how to 'get on with' whatever life holds for us. His indomitable spirit, his pleasure and delight in the world about him, have greatly enriched the lives of all of us who came into contact with him.

4 Hospital Based Projects

Early in 1981 another documentary film about mental handicap hospitals was shown on television. 'Silent Minority' presented scenes of the hospital in which Joey and his friends had spent most of their lives, and of Borocourt Hospital in Berkshire.

Viewing the situation from the outside, the producer and camera team saw little of the small daily acts which made some degree of homeliness possible even within the most inhospitable walls. Conditions which the television crew observed had a profound and shocking impact upon them, and their dismay was transferred to the presentation they made to the viewing public. 'Silent Minority' revealed conditions within *some* hospitals and brought into comfortable sitting rooms the plight of *some* mentally handicapped people, a subject of which many people had not previously been aware and which had been quite unknown to most of the population.

The hospital residents were portrayed as living in horrific conditions, herded into wired pens, naked and distressed. The impression given was that all hospitals had these conditions and that all patients lived in this way, which is far from true. It had the effect, however, of alerting the public to the urgent need for the community to provide alternative places for people to live and to provide the facilities for them to be trained to do so.

In the well-nigh hysterical reaction to the film which, like many such reactions, unfortunately died away fairly soon, it was not made clear how many hospitals of the kind had already made provision for their residents to move out into the community, nor how many different types of accommodation had been provided by a great many different routes. For example, one authority in Cumbria had decided to move out a considerable number of patients in small groups for retraining in a property some distance from the hospital, and then asked the local council to provide housing for them. Another authority in Plymouth had decided on a similar project, but managed to cooperate with a voluntary society and a housing association to provide the accommodation.

Projects designed to habilitate long-stay hospital residents for community living have been progressing in many different areas. Some examples have been studied for this book.

Plymouth, Devon

The Community Mental Handicap Service in Plymouth has been developed over the last four years and is planning for the future. Dr. Waters, Consultant Psychiatrist, acknowledges that the National Health Service, represented by the Area Health Authorities and Regional Hospital Boards, was not created to provide housing but to provide medical services which would prepare people and enable them to live in the community or to return to the community following hospital treatment; nevertheless, his appointment was the result of local pressure to improve *all* community based services for mentally handicapped people and was unique in that respect.

The Plymouth Plan is to create local geographical units linked with Community Teams, which would function as resource centres for each area and provide all the services required by mentally handicapped people and their families. They would only provide hospital residential places for patients in need of continuing treatment, or for short-term family relief services.

The following statement has been issued by the planning committee:

1. The Resource Centre Headquarters is currently at Wingfield Mansions and this Centre provides office accommodation for the senior professionals with specialist skills, so that they can be made available for the entire area.

2. There will be a residential unit, Cumberland House, to be filled by twenty patients from the Royal Western Coun-

ties Hospital, which will evolve into a Community Unit for South Plymouth.

3. A residential unit of ten places will be established at High-bury. Highbury House is the property of the Local Society who made available to the Department of Mental Handicap, Plymouth Health District, accommodation to facilitate the initial planning of the services and to allow some residential beds for ten to twelve persons as an emergency measure.

4. Two residential units, each accommodating ten children, are provided at Tamar House and Beckley Unit, Crownhill. The latter will ultimately provide twenty-five beds for patients who, after habilitation, can be discharged from the Royal Western Counties Hospital.

The primary concern of the Health Authority is the medical care of mentally handicapped people and the provision of services which would overcome their disabilities and enable them to be discharged from hospitalisation.

Experience has already been gained at Tamar House, a former Barnardo's Home on a council estate, which was offered to the Health Authority to house ten hospitalised children in the low ability range. Funds were extremely restricted; there were many administrative difficulties in transferring money from existing services to the new project, and the lack of financial support resulted in some changes to the plans originally made for the work of Tamar House. For example, the organisers had hoped to have individual catering and to provide a more homely atmosphere at meal-times, but they were forced to accept central catering supplied by the hospital services.

Great care was given to the selection of professional staff, as it was decided that the Service should spend the limited resources on the salaries of the right people for the job, rather than on expensive furniture and fittings.

The children came to Tamar House with the nursing staff from the hospital, so that they were familiar with those caring for them, and they were admitted in small groups of two or three at a time. Over the entire period only one boy had to be returned to the Royal Western Counties Hospital. It was thought that they would need a classroom on the site and this was accordingly set up for the first three months, but at the end of that time all the children were able to go out to classrooms at the Special School.

One major difficulty has been the inter-professional relationship between qualified nursing staff and qualified teachers at the school; both groups are unanimous in believing that programmes designed for education at the school must be continued by the nursing and care staff at home, but in practice it has proved very difficult for administrative reasons to achieve the full cooperation with the Education Authorities which would have enabled this to occur.

Permanent homes for mentally handicapped people, as opposed to rehabilitation units, should be provided by the Social Services Departments and voluntary societies, but Plymouth had only one adult hostel of seventeen places and no children's homes. Since the support services for mentally handicapped people must be constantly adjusted to their changing needs, it was recognised that a more flexible housing plan was urgently required. The Area Health Authority Survey in West Devon showed that 91% of mentally handicapped people were under forty years of age, 57% of these being women; these figures gave some indication of the future services which would be needed.

Housing Associations can work in cooperation with Local Authorities, and in Plymouth a good working partnership has been achieved with the Devon and Cornwall Housing Association. Funds for housing association work come from Central Government Housing Corporation or the Local Authority. In the past, housing associations provided in the main general family accommodation, and 50% of all places provided by them had to be offered to the Local Authority. (Details of a successful partnership with a housing association are given in the chapter on Local Authority Housing.)

In recent years there has been growing pressure on housing associations to provide for groups with special needs. Single workers, the elderly, both active and frail, ex-offenders, alcoholics and physically handicapped people can all now be offered homes within the general allocation, and mentally handicapped people can also be provided with housing if they are able to live independently, with the usual support from the Social Services Departments given to other disability groups.

The Plymouth project grew out of a situation in which nothing at all existed previously. It is still in a developing stage and will provide excellent opportunities for further study.

Aldingham, Cumbria

In contrast, the Aldingham project emerged from the sub-normality hospital, Dovenby Hall, which has just under four hundred residents.

In 1977 Dovenby Hall was faced with the need to close a ward in order that it might be upgraded, and staff were obliged to find alternative beds for sixty-four mentally handicapped male patients. Some were placed in other wards at Dovenby Hospital, and a search began for temporary accommodation for the remaining patients in other hospitals administered by the Regional Health Authority.

Two offers were received of huts in the grounds of older hospitals and were rejected as unsuitable. Finally, the hospital was offered Aldingham Hall, a large manor house which had been used as a convalescent home for surgical patients but had been run down and had stood empty for six months.

Aldingham Hall was situated sixty miles from Dovenby Hall and was isolated on a coastal road eight miles from Alveston, with a very poor local bus service. When the Dovenby Hall Hospital team visited Aldingham, they thought that it could have possibilities as a Habilitation Centre to which longstay patients from the hospital might be moved and prepared for community life. They asked staff at the hospital to nominate people they felt would profit by such a programme and ninety residents were nominated, all of whom were assessed by the clinical psychologist and by the ward staff.

All those chosen as a result of this process were taken to Aldingham and asked if they wished to be transferred there for the training programme. Some immediately decided they would prefer to remain in the familiar surroundings of the hospital. Thirty people were finally chosen and in April 1978 preliminary recruitment of staff began. Hospital staff were asked to volunteer to go to Aldingham, domestic and other helping staff were recruited from local people, and both the Education Authority and the Social Services agreed to supply staff for teaching and welfare. In addition, locally based volunteers were recruited to launch the project.

The first major hurdle was an objection from the local residents to the whole concept of using Aldingham Hall for this purpose, and a meeting of the Parish Council was called at which the Regional Authority District Administrator attempted to explain the project to the local residents. They, however, informed him that they intended to write to the County Council to demand that the project be abandoned. Since the joint consultative committee had already approved the scheme and funding, the decision could not be reversed but, nevertheless, the project started amid considerable distrust and resistance from the local people.

The first residents of Aldingham were sixteen men and fourteen women, their ages ranging from seventeen to sixty-five years. The time they had spent in Dovenby Hall varied from a minimum of seven years to a maximum of forty-nine years. The operational policy was to encourage independence in all the residents at all times, and to employ as many instructors and helpers with differing skills as possible, so as to create a homely atmosphere for all the residents. The ultimate objective was to move residents to permanent homes of their own, but when the experiment commenced there were no houses available to which they could be transferred. However, by the middle of 1978 a housing association had agreed to provide them with some accommodation.

Unfortunately, this first group home provided by the housing association actually fell down, while the people were living there. This setback was turned to advantage as, instead of accepting defeat and moving the residents back to Aldingham, or even to Dovenby Hall, it was decided to apply to the Local Authority to provide them with accommodation as homeless persons, and it was because of this policy that they were first established in temporary council accommodation in the city and later in council houses.

In October 1979 Aldingham acquired a shared property divided into flats for eight residents, five male and three female, which had individual bedrooms but shared kitchens and bathrooms, fridges, cookers, washing machines, etc., on each floor. This type of living has proved extremely beneficial and has an advantage over self-contained flatlets or bedsitters in that the residents can meet together and share facilities such as sitting-room and dining-room, while maintaining individual privacy, but are spared the loneliness which is often a concomitant of self-contained living.

This shared living, called 'cluster' flats, is currently provided by the Impact Housing Association and managed on a voluntary basis by MIND.

The scheme has continued to provide places in the community for mentally handicapped people who have passed through the Aldingham Hall Training Programme; one couple have married and now live in a council flat. The experiment was originally for one year only, but it is now being funded on a yearly renewal basis. One of the most interesting aspects of the teaching programme was that, from the moment residents entered Aldingham, no centrally prepared meal was provided; self-catering began immediately, with instructors or local helpers working alongside each individual and providing a model for imitation by the handicapped person.

Within a very short period of time the residents, divided into small groups of five with an equal number of helpers, were able to prepare simple meals for themselves for which they had shop-ped in the local town. The isolation of the Centre created a par-ticular difficulty in that their shopping had to be done between the bus service arrival and departure times, so that the educational value was limited to the actual purchase of items and could not be extended to allow for a period of choice or of longer social contact with other shoppers. The need to conclude their purchases quickly put the residents under some stress.

I have not heard this point made before, and I think it is a valuable one to bear in mind in the setting up of training programmes based on neighbourhood facilities.

The residents, who had previously had their drugs given to them under supervision by the trained staff, were all taught how to take a prescription to the chemist to receive their medicine, how to care for it safely and how to check that the dosage was correct. They were also given instruction in simple first-aid; for example, how to deal with an epileptic fit.

It is obvious that this experimental programme, forced on a subnormality hospital out of sheer necessity, has achieved some remarkable results, not only in its final objectives but in the multi-disciplinary teamwork by professionals from many different fields, and by instructional staff such as the gardener and cook, all of whom accepted an equal and sharing role. Their only directive was that they should not, themselves, perform the necessary tasks, but should be on hand to ensure that the residents could undertake the tasks, at first with help and, finally, completely independently.

Ashington, Morpeth, Northumberland

A report issued in June, 1981, describes a scheme to return severely mentally handicapped children from Northgate Hospital into the community in which their families live – Ashington, a small mining village.

The children concerned in the 1981 report were teenagers, with such severe disabilities that it would not appear that they could ever live outside the hospital. Two could not walk, three had no speech and four were not even able to communicate their need to use the lavatory. The Ashington house was run by three health authority staff, employed to do the shopping, cooking, laundry and housework, as well as to provide a 'sleep-in' supervision on a rota basis. All relevant medical services such as dental care, health visiting and district nursing were provided from the community services.

The report commences with a significant paragraph: 'The development of homes in Northumberland represents not only a move away from the traditional models of long-stay care for mentally handicapped people, but also a unique opportunity for the *reconciliation* of Health Authority and Social Services residential provision.'

Having utilised a four-bedroomed council house and made some small adaptations, the hospital was ready to commence this process of friendly liaison. The whole emphasis of the project was to create, as far as possible, the stability of a good family home in which the children could take a full part. The upper limit for entrance to this house was given as 18 years.

The report gives full details of the arrangements for staff, their salaries and duties, and the way in which the house is to be financed and maintained. Bank accounts at the Trustee Savings Bank will be opened in the name of each child resident and used for such personal expenditure as clothing, toys and hobbies, the responsible staff member rendering details of the accounts to the Area Treasurer of the Health Authority. Funds in these accounts can be augmented in case of need by allocations from the Area Treasurer.

It has been anticipated that the children in the home may receive money from other sources – families, friends and neighbours or charitable sources – as well as the state benefits to which they are entitled, and the AHA Treasurer has laid down very specific guidelines to ensure that such funds are used correctly and accounted for in a way acceptable to audit.

A home designed for children during their adolescent years cannot fall into my self-designed criteria of a 'home of their own', because the report states that children will be 'discharged' from the home and will 'move on to an Adult Training Centre' or 'the most suitable residential accommodation. This will be kept under constant review'. (But what residential accommodation, and where?)

This excellent and detailed report can be taken as a model of how young adults, severely and doubly handicapped, can live in an ordinary house with proper support. It covers the setting up of the project, the staff required, their daily programme of duty, the professionals needed in the assessment of the children and the review of their progress. Parents and families are to be free to visit at any time, while other visitors may come only on an invited basis, just as in an ordinary home.

The only thing missing from the report is a statement saying whether and on what terms those children, on reaching adult life, can continue to live in the home they have come to recognise as 'theirs', should they wish to remain there. Is the home envisaged as 'training' them to live as independently as possible, with the ultimate intention of moving them into different council houses and thus making room for others? Or is the scheme designed to enable them to achieve such a degree of independence that the support services, including the 'sleep-in' members of staff, are gradually withdrawn as the children become adults, until those able to live together as a group *are* living in a home of their own, supported by the community services available to their neighbours?

Some suggestions for the future are promised in the next report of the project.

The Wessex Experiment

One of the earliest community-based projects designed by a hospital authority was the setting up in 1970 of a scheme eventually to provide 450 places, in small community-based units, for children who would otherwise be expected to need permanent hospital care. Five of these, described as 'locally based hospital units' – four for children and one for adults, each comprising twenty to twenty-five places – were the subject of a controlled study and evaluation.

The idea of locally based units arose when the Western Regional Hospital Board was required to accept and plan for the residential care of all mentally handicapped people within the Regional Board's own boundaries, and it was decided to explore the feasibility of providing this accommodation in several small community units, rather than in a large mental handicap hospital.

The first two units were provided in Portsmouth and Southampton and received children from a selected geographical half of each city – children from the other half continuing to be admitted to hospital if they needed residential care. The hospital group was accommodated in villas within the hospital grounds and served as a control in the experiment.

One of the objects of the community-based project was to maintain the relationships with family and neighbourhood which were difficult to preserve when visits to a distant hospital were required.

The costs involved in the experiment were carefully monitored, in order to evaluate the desirability of using NHS funds for future units of this type, rather than devoting them to the maintenance and up-grading of existing hospitals. In a concise assessment of the experiment, the units are described as:

> relatively small places for twenty to twenty-five people, located in and serving a defined catchment area of town or city, designed to be as close as possible to a domestic, homely environment. The aim was for the mentally handicapped residents to share in the ordinary life of the community to which they belonged or had their closest kinship ties. In addition, it was considered that the major requirement of mentally handicapped people in residential care was for an alternative caring home, rather than for the treatment which is given in most establishments termed hospitals.

The necessity for a high ratio of staff to residents was anticipated, but nursing qualifications were not considered obligatory; in the event, however, the majority of senior staff were in fact trained nurses.

In accordance with the determination to preserve family links, visiting by relatives was totally unrestricted, and the resident children could be taken out by day or could stay overnight in their own homes. Relatives were encouraged to come in to the unit and to participate in the daily programme.

The project was designed from its inception as a research experiment and the behaviour of the residents was carefully recorded, as was that of the control groups remaining in hospital. A system of recording the activities throughout the day was devised and findings collected.

The evaluation showed that the children in the smaller units were more active and made more progress than the children in the hospital, and that the costs per child were comparable. Staff salaries accounted for a high percentage of the per capita costs, and a higher than average ratio must have been required to monitor the project to research standards.

Most interesting to me is the fact that there were four units designated for children, and only one for adults. This obviously reflected the situation in 1970 and '71 when *Better Services for the Mentally Handicapped* defined removing *children* from the wards of mental handicap hospitals as a primary objective.

The question arises, what is planned for these children when they become adults? I put this question to the Health Care Evaluation Research Team and quote from their reply:

The four units designed for children continue to have the same role, i.e. they serve the residential needs of people from birth to age 16–18 years. On reaching this age children are transferred to other forms of care. In many cases this has meant readmission to traditional large hospitals, in some, return to the family home and in some, admission to similar local units for adults. Unfortunately, the provision of local homes for adults has only recently become more common. There is still a long way to go, as most District authorities have given priority to providing local homes for children; as the same number of homes is required for adults as is needed to serve each group of children, the unsatisfactory situation here is likely to persist for some time yet. However, Wessex Region formulated a ten-year plan for 1979–89 to complete local provision, so that by the end of this decade there is the expectation that people who require residential care at any stage of their lives can receive it in a local facility.

Following the original development of locally-based homes in Wessex, the residential care section of the research team has begun to look at the provision of smaller units using ordinary housing. At the moment, one eight-place home for severely and profoundly mentally handicapped adults has been provided and a further one is due to open. They are both in Andover and are the first of the planned provision by Winchester Health District in response to Wessex Region's proposal to provide comprehensive services in each Health District during this decade.

The present situation is frankly described by the Team as 'unsatisfactory'. If forward planning does not take into account the inevitable bottle-neck situation which is bound to arise if no on-ward movement is considered from residences designed only for childhood, this unsatisfactory situation will continue.

Not only the future of those in the population at present must be planned for, but of those who will be born in this decade. The planned provision for the future cannot be considered in the finite terms of a certain number of units, but as a percentage of all housing stock available from all sources. A home for life must still be the major objective, but the common problems of increasing age and its disabilities make it necessary for provision in local schemes for the elderly to include some mentally handicapped residents also.

The ten-year plan quoted provides for a final total of thirteen units of eight beds each for adults, and only one new unit to be provided in 1990 specifically for children, thus accepting the principle of care in the family home for most mentally handicapped children as the desirable norm. It further states that only twenty-six children in the total population of over 100,000 are expected to be in need of special services (1985 prediction) and that a unit currently providing eighteen places for children has vacant places today. This would suggest that children, even those with severe handicaps, are now being cared for at home; in the future, schemes designed to provide alternatives for the young adult may well replace plans for children's residences, enabling them to leave the family home for more independent living.

The plan acknowledges this in the concluding analysis of costs, and implies that the Health and Social Services intend to use capital to acquire homes from other sources than local authority housing, stating that to provide the required places there will be 'maximum concentration on finding favourable sites/buildings in one locality and continuous liaison with local estate agents'.

The revenue costs of the whole project include a large element for staff salaries. Certainly staff will be needed in the early preparation stages and for support as the residents settle in, but experience elsewhere seems to suggest that units of ordinary housing with a smaller group of people, four or less, require only a modest staff establishment, non-resident, to give the help needed.

Investigation of current projects reveals a fascinating diversity of approach, the effect of local conditions and traditional attitudes held by local people towards their neighbours.

The courtesy of so many authorities in supplying details of their own experience and of their forward planning, makes possible informed study of current projects. All those concerned can see demonstrated the results of projects initiated as long ago as ten or more years. Those who have recorded the various schemes have not hesitated to record their mistakes, as well as the factors which contribute to success.

5 Future Plans for Hospitals

Of the patients remaining in mental handicap hospitals, numbering around 40,000 or so in 1982, probably at least half are capable of living independently outside, if community schemes can be provided. I say 'schemes' advisedly, for there are many elements to consider in the movement of hospital residents.

Conditions within the hospital need to be carefully structured and monitored if the programme is to be designed for eventual discharge.

The principle of self-selected groups means that residents need the opportunity to choose their friends; they should not be restricted to forming friendships only with those in their immediate proximity. In the course of my visits I heard several times of residents in community homes who regretted the loss of a particular friend, sometimes from another ward. It is possible that staff did not know of the bond between these particular patients.

If people are selected for preparation and training solely on the grounds of their relatively equal standard of ability, so that a group can be more easily taught together; or if they are chosen because they have had the apparently common experience of always sharing the same ward; or if similarity of temperament is the criterion – then the project is still being staff-designed, rather than self-determined by mentally handicapped people themselves. When they move out they may no longer have the same staff supporting them. The organised routine of hospital life may well have obscured their real and individual needs and suppressed personality traits, both positive and negative, which will affect the way they adapt as a group to life outside.

During a visit to a group of people living in a council house, I met a young woman who expressed violent objections to having been nominated to appear in a television documentary without prior consultation. She was obviously outgoing and extrovert, and active to a degree that would have presented very real problems in a hospital ward where her need for self expression and attention would have resulted in 'acting-up' scenes; probably the staff concerned had genuinely felt that she would welcome the opportunity to express her feelings to a wider audience. She might well have done so, but her objection, that it was *their* choice, not hers, was valid; it demonstrates that the ultimate success of any hospital project will depend upon how carefully and accurately the selection of a group has been made. It shows, too, how important it is to consult the mentally handicapped people themselves before arriving at any decision.

Methods of training vary from place to place. Residents may receive initial preparation in the hospital itself, from staff they know well, working with other instructors with special skills, for example, in cookery; or they may go out to centres where these skills are taught.

It is also important to distinguish between the acquisition of practical skills: cookery, housekeeping, hygiene, clothing, using money, using the telephone, and all the hundred and one amenities of life today; and the skills of living together with others: dealing with arguments, the relative dominance within a group, the roles which each member will play at different times.

Some of the simple skills can be learnt anywhere, but since so many of the more difficult skills of shared living can only be learnt by experience, there is probably a good case to be made for learning the domestic skills from the start, in company with one's future companions and in the place that will be one's home. If hospital preparation and selection is not possible, then a transition residence will be needed, and it may be that this is the function of the hostel. However, it can only be designated a 'training hostel' or 'training home', if there is already a planned home to move *to*; one cannot remain in training for ever, with no concrete goal in sight to give purpose to the whole exercise.

There will also be a need for a variety of homes for those who, after living with a group, large or small, decide that the time has come for them to branch out and live alone, or with one other person. Among hospital residents these will probably be the younger people, but older residents may still prefer bed-sitting rooms in a house which has a resident staff person, to sharing a home with three or four friends.

It is to be hoped that better support services will eventually enable mentally handicapped young children, and those unborn today, to live permanently with their own families, but there may well be a place for the slightly larger residence as well. Catering for groups of no more than eight children, with an appropriate number of staff, it would provide accommodation for education facilities during the school week, for needed short respite breaks for parents, or for family crises. At present parental emergencies too often mean hospitalisation for the child.

A hospital will still be needed for those requiring intensive medical care, but not a mental handicap hospital. Skilled nursing, even for chronically disabled people, can be provided with humanity and dignity in much smaller units than we are currently obliged to use. Perhaps the idea of a hospice for the terminally ill could be adapted for the few severely and profoundly physically and mentally handicapped, and would be staffed by those who have a genuine vocation for such work; while the even smaller number of mentally handicapped people who are doubly afflicted with mental illness can already be cared for in the psychiatric hospitals.

For the remaining, and much larger number, a properly designed plan of community care is long overdue.

In St. Lawrence's Hospital, where Joey and his friends lived for so long, very few of the patients are there as the result of a committal order; most are voluntary patients, and, theoretically, they are free to leave. They receive personal allowances which are banked in their individual names and may only be used for their personal benefit. These accounts are held by the Health Authority's Accounts Department. Every resident has an individual record of payments in and out.

Dr. Geoffrey Harris says there is something like two-to-three hundred thousand pounds sitting in deposit accounts in Croydon because patients have so few opportunities to spend their money, and the staff are working desperately around this. One of the answers may be the formation of clubs to which subscriptions are made, the club then deciding how to spend the money. But administration and auditors insist that the spending has to be personal. The purchase of something for the ward, like buying a music centre, cannot be done from 'pooled' money.

If there are two hundred people who are *entitled* to a mobility allowance, for example, the hospital will claim it for them even if they are not going to be able to spend it easily. Much extra money is coming in now, and much of it remains unused because very few can spend it independently. For example, in order to take residents out, the staff would need to order taxis and make special arrangement, so creating additional problems.

The experience of setting up the scheme for Little Holland Village in the grounds of St. Lawrence's Hospital, and the resources available to the residents, make it plain, at least to me, that the often repeated objection to community living – financial cost – is totally misunderstood. A changed use of the funds currently being spent in dozens of different directions, would provide ample resources for expert professional staff, medical and educational, at appropriate periods in the lives of mentally handicapped people, as well as a place for them to live. It is a matter of utilising the resources of the community which are available to the rest of us.

Geoffrey Harris feels that many large hospitals have much more land than they can ever use, particularly down in the south. This is how he sums up his very personal view of the way the present situation should change:

When I started the project, I was not aware, as I am now, of all the politics and the way people feel. I thought we were doing something really new and really good and I was very pleased. I was brought down to earth and a bit deflated, as time went on, when people came and said 'Yes, lovely bungalows but why are they *here*?' Fair enough, the Development Team said more or less the same thing. I do not know now if we ever will get the twelve bungalows we had planned for. If people are so anti-hospital that even building on hospital ground is taboo, we shall not get any more money, but I shall go on trying to get more bungalows; there are people still in the wards for whom the only hope of a real home is in one of our bungalows, with full hospital support.

There might be some people who do not need permanent resident staff but who would need a careful measure of super-vision, and others who might need resident staff as well. There will still be some left who need a hospital *type* of care. If they are to be cared for in the outside community it will need something of the same *pattern* of care as present hospitals offer but not in the present type of building. It could mean building a new type of hostel in the community that is designed to take people of a high level of dependence.

If I have any vision of what the future might be, it is that the bungalows could last and become part of the Caterham com-munity – even if you knock the rest of the Hospital down.

6 Conclusions

From frequent visits to St. Lawrence's Hospital and the experience gained in setting up Little Holland Village, from discussions in connection with that project and with other hospital schemes, the message is clear. There can be no one *national* solution.

Hospitals like St. Lawrence's which have long received residents mainly from one area will have local considerations to consider. Areas which have despatched their mentally handicapped residents to distant hospitals and are now anxious to reclaim them will have different problems. Housing availability in the hard-pressed inner cities will be different from less populated rural areas.

The whole scheme of hospital training involves setting up, within a hospital, training units which correspond to those where people will be required to live when they leave the hospital. It also requires that the people who are to train them have personal experience of community living. Nowadays very few members of staff have spent their entire adult lives inside the hospital, but this is still the case in many of the large corrective institutions, and the training for community life is not likely to be effective if it is carried out by people who are themselves institutionalised by the system.

Small independent units can be established within hospital grounds, but will require links with the community from the start. Initially such a scheme may be an expensive exercise, but probably not more than the cost of upgrading existing wards and converting them into hostels. There is the additional advantage that if suitably designed and sited, such small units may well remain to add to the community housing stock after the outmoded institution has been demolished. In the main, homes for mentally handicapped people are ordinary houses, provided by the local authority or by a housing association. What is needed in addition is effective support.

The experiences described in the preceding chapters reveal many important factors. First, the vital importance of the key person to initiate, to persevere, and then to delegate responsibility for the scheme. Secondly, the need for selection and training of all concerned, both staff and residents, and for adequate time to prepare for the transfer; and thirdly, and most importantly, the true realisation that mentally handicapped people are *people* first, and handicapped as a secondary attribute.

It is immediately apparent that almost all groups can only function in the outside world if the group is made up of people with complementary skills. For example, if there is one member of the group whose intelligence is slightly above that of the others but who is, perhaps, physically disabled, that person will need to have, within this small family group, people with sufficient physical ability to help him or her.

Different innate gifts are equally necessary. There are those who have a gift for housekeeping, and there are those who have a gift for gardening and there are those who have the methodical type of mind to work, for example, stacking shelves in a supermarket. There is also the matter of emotional temperament, and it is absolutely clear that when the groups are set up they must be, as far as is humanly possible, self-selected. In other words, they must be groups of *friends*, people who have already come to terms with the differences in their temperament and who are able to live together, making allowances for the individual needs of each.

Some of the mistakes which have been made in the arbitrary selection of people as living companions resulted in emotional stress and in considerable difficulties which could have been avoided.

Another arrangement which has been tried is to bring together a mixed group of people from different backgrounds. A few hospital residents are chosen to set up home with one or two other people who have not previously lived in subnormality hospitals; having already acquired some of the skills of living in the community, these people have valuable experience to pass on to the hospital group.

At this moment there are many hospitals actively training patients to live in the community, in sharp contrast to the situation a few years ago when people were hurtled out of longstay hospitals into the community without any training or preparation, and who became exploited by seedy boarding houses and other similar establishments. There is a large volume of experience now on the whole problem of moving into some type of community living patients who have been accustomed to living in large subnormality hospitals and who, in many cases, are totally unprepared for life outside. Many mistakes have been made, but they have served to pinpoint the most pressing needs in order to prevent similar errors in planning and make provision for the future.

We must find a method of ensuring that when a home is provided for mentally handicapped people it is, within reason, a home for life. If their circumstances change, obviously it may be necessary for them to have some kind of alternative accommodation, but once removed from an institution they should not be forced to enter it again for reasons that are not medical.

Even residents, long institutionalised and advancing in years, can acquire new skills if they are taught practically and patiently by instructors prepared to allow them to make mistakes. The three friends of Joey Deacon all learned the skills necessary to care for a profoundly handicapped man, and looked after him with only minimum supervision, while cooking and carrying out domestic tasks they had never performed before.

Residents from Dovenby Hall were literally forced, as homeless persons, into community living, and managed it well because of the planned educational programme which had preceded it. In Plymouth, spurred by the Local Society for Mentally Handicapped Children, a new appointment was made through the NHS, to provide a new and enlightened service to the community.

Throughout the country there are examples of such projects which demonstrate the determination and understanding of the staff of large mental handicap hospitals to help the patients in their care into independent living. Their efforts are doomed unless suitable homes are provided into which these people can move.

We may all find that these less able people among us, by their example of care for each other, help us to re-learn the lesson that we are not isolated each from each, and that the community is both responsible for and enriched by the duty of concern for the needs of others.

PART TWO

Preparing to Leave the Family Home

1 The First Steps to Independence

The Historical Background

Traditionally, the largest group of mentally handicapped people has comprised those living at home with their own families. For them the provision of a home of their own has often never been considered, especially if the handicapped member of the family was born years ago, at a time when no help or support service was available. Some of these people, of both sexes, have achieved a remarkable degree of self-care in their own familiar surroundings. Many of them contribute significantly to the comfort and independence of their now aged parents. Some are able to shop and use public transport and carry out household duties. These are the children of parents who, without specialist knowledge, nevertheless patiently and practically helped their handicapped child to develop his potential abilities to the full.

Others of this older age-group, often more severely handicapped, are totally dependent on parents and other family members. As their brothers and sisters move away from home, the anxiety of the parents for the future of the handicapped son or daughter becomes an increasing nightmare.

Until recently, little help or advice was available to those who gave birth to a mentally handicapped child. Many parents were told when their children were born that they would always be dependent upon them and unable to care for themselves, and would be in constant danger of exploitation. This advice was often given in good faith; little was known at that time of the possible development which could be achieved by individual programmes of education.

So the prophecy of total dependency fulfilled itself. Education in Junior Training Centres, run by the Local Health Department, was followed by daily attendance at Adult Training

Centres, where simple light industrial tasks filled the day for the young adults, and continued as a pattern into advancing age.

Many of these centres were on the outskirts of town, some on industrial sites, and this meant that trainees were collected from their homes by bus and returned at the end of the day by the same means. They were thus effectively isolated from their neighbours. At the weekends, parents often continued the isolating process – unconsciously accepting the fact that their sons and daughters were different from others, needed more supervision, should not have relationships with the opposite sex and could not be expected to develop beyond the level at which they had ceased their early training.

Not all Training Centres were run on such pessimistic lines. Some managers already knew that many of their trainees had a capacity for development beyond what was expected and were anxious to widen the scope of activities to achieve greater independence. Sometimes their efforts were misinterpreted by the parents, who still saw themselves as ultimately responsible for the actions of their mentally handicapped sons and daughters, well beyond the age at which they were legally adult – at that time twenty-one years of age.

Even as late as the mid-sixties, the general public knew very little about mental handicap, and even less about what was done in the large isolated subnormality hospitals in which some adult mentally handicapped people had spent a lifetime. The greater proportion of the less severely handicapped still lived at home and continued to live at home well past the age when other young adults had left their parents to enter employment, marry and have homes of their own. In any community, their numbers were small, and as they attended special schools, or Junior Training Centres, in their childhood years, they were already isolated, even in their own neighbourhoods, and remained so as they grew older. On the death of their parents, most were received into hospital care for the rest of their lives.

But the attitudes of society were changing. In the 1960s a relaxation of standards of sexual behaviour meant that many young people began to live together outside marriage; the age of majority was lowered to eighteen years; responsibility for the actions of their children was gradually being removed from parents. These shifting attitudes placed the parents of mentally handicapped children in an acute dilemma. They knew, or thought they knew, the limits of independence to which their children could aspire. Many of them, for example, had never allowed their sons and daughters to cook a meal for themselves, or to travel on public transport.

The Slough Project
In 1960, The National Society for Mentally Handicapped Children (now granted a Royal Charter) announced to its 40,000 members a pilot scheme that would enable young adults to live away from home, in hostel accommodation, and to receive training for employment. A purpose-built unit was designed and sited in Slough, and opened to day trainees in 1962. In her excellent report upon the project, *The Mentally Handicapped Adolescent*, Dr. Eileen Baranyay describes it accurately as a 'child of its time'.

The prosperity and optimism of the 'Swinging Sixties' provided the climate to support innovation, while full employment led to the expectation that mentally handicapped people could, after appropriate training, secure work in the open job market. The major objective of Slough was to demonstrate that the trainees could produce work of marketable value under industrial conditions, and the unit's well equipped workshops offered the chance of a range of industrial skills.

In addition, there were residential hostel places for fifteen young men and fifteen young women, in single and double rooms, with shared sitting and dining rooms.

The experience of living away from home was an added bonus since many of the young people had not previously lived completely away from their families. Most returned for a weekend visit at least once a month, some more frequently.

Some, on arrival, needed help with shaving, bathing and dressing, and many had communication difficulties. Young people who have not been given sufficient incentives to speak and express themselves so that they are understood outside the family circle have a primary need in this area. Those who are familiar with mentally handicapped children often anticipate their needs, and by interpreting gestures or facial movements, quickly supply what is wanted. It takes time and patience to insist on the use of commonly understood speech.

The experience at Slough, where the young trainees were in daily contact with many different people – instructors, domestic staff and a constantly changing band of volunteers, including pupils from local schools – proved that when the need for speech arose, the facility in many cases rapidly improved. Getting on with other people, accepting discipline, learning skills, were all an integral part of the training.

In conjunction with the structured industrial work, the young people were also taught some domestic and housekeeping skills. They were free to make an evening cup of tea or milk drink, and were welcomed into the kitchens at the end of their working day, where they observed and helped with the chores of catering for a large group.

They were instructed in bed-making and were responsible for the tidiness of their own rooms, and at weekends, when no outside cleaning staff were employed, they helped to maintain order in the shared sitting-rooms, as well as in the dining-room and kitchens. They were also instructed in the use of simple household appliances such as the vacuum cleaner and electric iron. The young men who needed to shave learned to use electric razors.

Visiting local shops for sweets or fish and chips introduced the use of money and public transport and, later, sometimes with a note to the shopkeeper, they purchased articles of clothing of their own choice.

It became evident very soon that, with the major objective of training for work carried out through a full five-day week from 9 am to 5 pm, there was not sufficient time for concentrated instruction which could lead to independent living in a home of their own. There was a real need for leisure pursuits, for relaxation in a sport or hobby of their own choice. Many of the young trainees were tired at the end of the working day and less inclined to spend the free weekends in additional instruction.

This problem was exacerbated by the fact that the group contained a wide range of handicap. Some were so severely handicapped that they completely lacked motivation and would sit motionless until instructed, relapsing again when their task was complete.

Nevertheless, the Slough project was a landmark in the progression from isolation in the family home or hospital to community living.

The young people were living with others of the same age and similar interests. They had an element of choice in their use of leisure, of friendship and clothing. The trainees in the workshop were not all resident in the hostels, the thirty boarders being augmented by the original twenty day trainees. The staff were resident, each hostel having house parents who worked as instructors, cooks and housekeeping staff. Social training teachers were non-resident.

The nature of the scheme dictated the character of the training. It was a community with a homely atmosphere, not a training centre providing individual programmes for independent living. The acceptance of severely handicapped young people, some with an IQ of only 30, would have made the instruction and preparation of the trainees for living without support a mammoth task.

After training, which could be for a period of up to two years, most returned to their family homes, or to hostels in their own areas. The detailed report on the project and the case studies given by Eileen Baranyay in *The Mentally Handicapped Adolescent*, provide a vivid account of the achievements and also reflect contemporary attitudes towards the potential abilities of mentally handicapped people, classified at that time as 'ineducable', that is, with IQs of below 50. Several more years were to pass before the Education Act, 1971, conferred the right to appropriate education upon all mentally handicapped children. Meanwhile, Slough was receiving those deemed to be incapable of instruction, and was proving the classification 'ineducable' to be fallacious.

The interest aroused by the work at Slough, and the many possibilities it opened, focused attention on three new establishments set up for training by the Society in the years between 1965–67. Dilston Hall, Lufton Manor and Pengwern Hall each received young people for training in social skills, life skills and vocational skills, and offered a period of change from school, family and institutional life. Pengwern Hall has particularly concentrated on training for residence in a home of one's own.

The understanding that adolescence provided a second chance to make up for deficiencies of childhood education was becoming more widely accepted, and resulted in many innovative projects, both statutory and voluntary.

In this climate, the three MENCAP residential training establishments provided a chance of living away from home, combined with education and training. Unemployment was not yet a problem, and the chance of work in municipal horticultural activities, on the land or in shops and light industry was still possible. The philosophy in each of the three training centres was designed to increase independence and to develop the potential of the young mentally handicapped men and women who were accepted for training.

Pengwern Hall is studied next in some detail, as an example of what can be achieved with imagination and local cooperation.

2   Pengwern Hall

Pengwern Hall is situated in Rhuddlan, a few miles from Rhyl in the beautiful North Wales coastal area. The major industry of the area is agriculture, and there is seasonal tourism. Unemployment is higher than the national average, so that the establishment at Pengwern, accommodating residents, also provides welcome employment for local people who have been closely associated with the Hall for many years. It was previously a convalescent home.

The cooperation of the local community has therefore been more enthusiastic than in an amenity which is suddenly sited in a settled urban area. Goodwill on the part of neighbours is essential if any project involving mentally handicapped people is to be successful, and this goodwill must be actively and sensitively sought.

The opportunity for the trainees to learn a greater degree of independent living soon became possible at Pengwern by virtue of the availability, within the Hall complex, of some derelict buildings which it was possible to convert into small units. These units, plus the development of a structured programme of independence training, led, years later, to the occupation of houses in the community outside, at some distance from Pengwern Hall.

Martin Weinberg, the Director of Pengwern, has described how the project took shape and developed into the successful and wide-ranging scheme it is today:

> On the initial training course we had twenty youngsters who came from various parts of the United Kingdom as the result of a small information sheet which I sent out to a few local authority departments. This experimental period taught us all

that, even within a restricted period of three months, we could achieve a good deal. We didn't sit down and design a grand plan; we didn't even, in those days, come to a conclusion about where our efforts would lead.

What we actually learned from the youngsters who came and what we learned about the direction in which they developed, was that adolescence provides the best possible learning opportunity for independence. Within the home environment these movements towards adolescence were creating problems, as they invariably do in any normal home. The problems were increased by the fact that the efforts towards independence were being frustrated by lack of opportunity and the accepted dependent role within their families.

We started with one habitable building, the main Hall, and then embarked on the conversion of the coach-house block. Our initial thought about it was that we would make it into extra dormitory accommodation, but our experience had shown us that the youngsters we were providing for were capable of doing more for themselves; so we rethought our plan for the block and decided we would convert it into a row of normal houses which we hoped would give us the opportunity to train the youngsters to cope for themselves with all the basic activities of life.

The way in which we went about the conversion of the block was dictated to us by the need for funds. We had to find the money ourselves, so we started a number of fund-raising activities here at Pengwern. We had regular whist drives – North Wales is a place where people enjoy whist drives – and we had about 200 people coming every week. The young residents organised and catered for these events. We had local garden fêtes and we were given the use of shops in neighbouring towns, which we could run for a week or a couple of weeks, selling jumble or whatever came our way.

At the same time we were publicising our efforts and the conversion project through all local organisations.

This brought in many local people who came to our events, and they seemed to look kindly on what we were doing. We started getting support from many local organisations. Nobody gave us large sums of money, but lots of people gave us small amounts, and as the money came in we embarked on the work of converting the coach house and stable block.

In those early days we were fortunate to gain the assistance of a local builder who happened to be married to one of the staff at Pengwern. He came up at weekends and we saw that he got on very well with the trainees. So when we started to get enough funds together and the conversion of the block became a serious activity, we offered him a permanent post on the staff as a building instructor. He, together with the trainees and the help of our unskilled staff, converted the first coach house. That gave us the opportunity to think in terms of making our first steps towards independence training.

In time, the whole coach house and stable block was converted into a terrace of five four-bedroomed houses, in each of which six people lived with two house parents. At first, each house was a single-sex dwelling, but as the experimental phase passed, it was found that mixed sex units functioned much better, the different complementary abilities of the boys and girls making for simpler running of each house.

The idea of mixed sex units was very new at that time, and gave rise to the sort of anxieties often felt by parents who are contemplating a move into community care, where the supervision of social workers and house parents will replace the careful protection of home life.

One member of staff I talked to, on a visit to Pengwern, did express some personal anxieties. He was worried about the possibility of having a very susceptible, impressionable girl as one of his residents; even talking to her and passing over what advice he felt he could give without impressing his own moral values, might still leave her at risk. For him, anyway, there was at least a hypothetical dilemma as to whether he or a female member of staff should say, 'We can cope with everything about this girl, but we can't protect her from sexual exploitation'.

Martin Weinberg's response to such a situation was that any member of staff expressing that kind of concern would be speaking like any normal parent about his own daughter; and that if he wasn't able to express concern, or was not aware of the possibilities, he would be less valuable as a member of staff. He felt that living 'like other people' meant an acceptance of some of the risks of such living.

I first visited Pengwern Hall in 1970, at the time when the decision to convert the first range of derelict coach houses had been taken. The Hall was the only residential unit in use at that time. There, over thirty school-leavers, boys and girls of greatly varying ability, were undergoing residential training in social skills and independence. The name used for the course was 'transitional'. It was indeed a transition from the sheltered, completely protected life of home and special school, to a new environment, living closely with a group of strangers and learning new skills.

At this time the length of the course was designed to be three months, but some extension was possible if it was felt that the students would benefit. The main activities on the vocational side were horticultural; there was a large greenhouse in good order, and more than twenty acres of land surrounding the Hall. Market gardening was a major activity, and many of the young people returned home to obtain employment in this field.

On the day of my first visit I walked from the Hall to the coach house development, then in its first stage. An experienced builder was directing the activities of a group of young men and women amid the usual chaos of any building site. I have never forgotten the loving care with which one girl was patiently trowelling cement over an area designed to form the entrance to the house, nor the gentle supervision with which the builder watched her efforts. He, or any of the instructors, could have completed the task in a tenth of the time and with much greater efficiency. It requires a very special gift to be able to watch someone else painfully achieve a skill which you possess. At that moment I fully appreciated the magnitude of the task that the whole staff of Pengwern Hall had set for themselves, and their total dedication to it.

When, some years later, I saw that same derelict building

occupied and providing a warm comfortable home for a small 'family' unit, I was sharply reminded of the group of young people who had made those first pioneer steps in proving what could be done by mentally handicapped people, given the opportunity to learn and contribute to a project.

The residents of each house received a housekeeping allowance and shopped and cooked for themselves. The whole scheme was so successful that a further development was decided upon. An old school building at Llansannan was acquired, originally as a leisure centre to provide adventure training courses for young people living at the Hall. It is now being converted to provide another twelve-place residential unit.

The next venture was the conversion of a pair of semi-detached Victorian houses in St. Asaph – the tiny cathedral city two miles from Pengwern Hall – and the stage achieved at present, in 1982, includes a house in the main street of Rhuddlan, where a group of girls live with one resident staff member.

On my last visit, in Autumn 1981, I chatted to the young people now resident in the coach houses, all of whom are having their first taste of some degree of independence. They have resident house parents who help them to plan the daily menus – all have a chance to ask for their favourite foods – and to shop for the ingredients and to cook and serve them.

The young people had just returned from the mid-term break, spent at home with their families, and were showing photographs and gifts to each other. A party was being planned and they were all involved in the preparations. The coach house, which I had seen as a gutted shell of a building, was now a very comfortable, warm home. The only small difference from any ordinary house, which I observed in every residence I visited, was an exceptionally large and well-appointed kitchen. This room was obviously the hub of the house. The menu, patiently written by one of the residents, was pinned up on the dresser, and both boys and girls were engaged in tidying the house. All had extra personal laundry to do because they had been on holiday. The resident house parents were involved in all the activities, but so unobtrusively that I had some difficulty in identifying them among their charges.

Bedrooms reflected the personalities of their occupants. Wall posters, favourite soft toys, pot plants, records and all the usual clutter of adolescent living, were evidence that the little house was a real home. One of the girls had proved difficult to fit in with this group and a suggestion had been made that she should return to the Hall for a further period. Another girl had immediately offered to share her own room with the 'difficult' member, to see if they could get on together and so avoid the move back.

In each of the converted coach houses and stable block residences everyone was involved in making beds, washing up after breakfast, cleaning rooms and preparing for lunch. There was an informal bustle, but no muddle.

I then visited the small city of St. Asaph and waited in the corner shop, run by Pengwern Hall, for my hostess from the houses in the town. The shop was already busy with customers, and the resident staff manager was supervising the young people who were serving. The shop sells everything: vegetables, fruit, dairy foods, frozen food, canned and packeted products. An unusual feature is that they can serve very small quantities – a quarter pound of butter, for example – and as many of the customers I saw were elderly, there is no doubt that this is appreciated. The young people needed very little help from the staff member, but she usually checked the scales to ensure any goods were accurately weighed. The customers, including young mothers with babies, obviously used the shop as a social meeting place, as the old village shop used to provide in the past. One customer left a purchase behind on the counter, and one of the young trainees immediately set off to search the neighbouring shops in order to return it to her.

A young resident from the nearby houses arrived soon afterwards and conducted me to the terraced house where she lived. Two adjoining properties have been acquired at the end of a row of substantially built Victorian properties, and each of these has a group of mixed sex residents and house parents.

Everyone here was equally busy, but it was mainly the girls

who were at home. The boys had various local jobs and went out to them daily. The premises had needed little adaptation, but the large kitchen/dining room was again a feature. Good utility rooms and laundry rooms had also been added, and the same individuality was apparent in the bedrooms as in the coach houses.

The young residents were happy to show me round their homes, without the intervention of the staff, and explained their choice of meals. It is obviously a good thing that they all have a chance to select their preferences – my guide said that one of the group would eat baked beans all week, given the chance.

They are encouraged to go into Rhuddlan at least weekly to shop for major items, as it is thought that this presents better learning experience than to go to their own corner shop, where several of them work for a period during the day.

After visiting the bookshop, due to open the next day, I was welcomed by the four boys who live in a flat over another retail shop in the town centre. They look after themselves, cook and clean, but they have some supervision from staff next door and, while I was there, were having coffee made by one of the girl trainees who was paying a social visit, before the young men left for work.

Most of the young men are employed in the various horticulture and building conversion work connected with the Pengwern projects and are out of the houses for a good part of the day. In addition, some of them work in the Parks and Gardens Department of the Local Authority, while others assist at a local trout farm. Some of the residents of St. Asaph have moved on to the High Street house in Rhuddlan and come back daily by bus to their employment in St. Asaph.

The conversion work at Llansannan School was proceeding apace during my visit there. Several young men were at work under the supervision of the building instructors, and over the road, in the house which had once been the home of the headmaster, another group of young people, with the houseparent, were preparing for the midday meal.

The impression of homely family living in every residence, the evident pleasure shown by all the young people in having visitors to offer hospitality, and to share their pride in their possessions, is sufficient evidence of the success of this particular project.

Following my visits to the residences, Martin Weinberg gave me his views on the development of the Pengwern experiment, and his thinking behind the work of preparing young people for true independence, to the limit of each individual's ability:

> Respect for the mentally handicapped person as an individual implies acceptance of the need to make mistakes, to differ from others without violent behaviour, to express personal likes and dislikes, in short, to be responsible for the results of behaviour, however painful the process.
>
> The young people at Pengwern are a cross-section of the physically able mentally handicapped. Some are extremely competent, others less so. In their residential situation they have a choice of those who will live with them, and daily practice in adapting their wishes to those of others. They share, also, in the daily hazards which affect us all, for real life is not free from dangers and distress, and true life preparation must take this into account.

Preparation will certainly be needed for young people who have always lived at home. No matter how competent they become in household management, in handling money and other amenities, such as the telephone and public transport, they will still need actual practical experience of sharing a home with strangers and achieving a degree of happiness.

At the moment, training schemes like those at Pengwern often involve leaving the family and the familiar district. I asked Martin Weinberg if he felt that this separation from the known environment was a positive factor in the success of the training. He agreed that it was a very big step for the young people, and that they naturally had a great deal of adjustment to make to it, but in his view the really great step must be taken by the parents; their difficulty lay in accepting that the separation for training was only the first stage in a process designed to prepare both parent and child for the fact that they would not live together for ever.

Pengwern has attempted to help young people who have been

resident in hospitals, but in the main this group has proved to be beyond the caring capacity of the staff. Most have such severe behaviour problems that they constitute a danger both to themselves and others. Martin Weinberg feels that long stay hospital patients also suffer a massive loss of self-confidence, having always accepted that the professional staff would make decisions for them and would know what was best for them; this attitude makes even small steps into independence much more difficult to achieve. If young people have lived at home during childhood, they have a much better chance of achieving independence than if they have spent years in and out of hospitals or resident homes.

Martin Weinberg involves all the staff in every aspect of the daily routine, using each situation as a teaching experience. The young residents learn by example and daily practice how to look after themselves and their homes; every contact becomes an opportunity for learning and is fully exploited to improve communication and the social skills of getting on with others. The emphasis upon meal-preparation, shown by the large, well equipped kitchens, and by the involvement of the residents in the planning, shopping and cooking, is an example of the teaching of basic skills. As Martin Weinberg says, 'Everyone is interested in food; we always concentrate on the things that will arouse interest and achieve cooperation, so cooking and eating together provide a first-class learning situation.'

3 Conclusions

If mentally handicapped children are no longer to be admitted to hospitals as a routine procedure, but are to be cared for at home by their families with appropriate support, their future after leaving school needs urgent consideration. Already the old concepts of the role of the Adult Training Centre – as an industrial training agency, providing a work simulated environment – are being questioned. Many Adult Centres now provide a planned programme of self-help and social skill training on an individual basis, designed as far as possible to equip each person for adult life. But although these young people, living at home, receive training in all areas of community life, many have no chance of practising their skills outside their own homes.

The education service, until 1971 concerned only with mentally handicapped pupils with an IQ of over 50, now provides education for even the severely educationally handicapped. The tragedy is, however, that after ten years' experience in this field, it is sending young adults of sixteen to nineteen years out into a world which is still not prepared to carry on the work which the schools have begun. The need of these youngsters for continued education should not condemn them to become life-long students, with no future but daily attendance at a 'centre' of some kind.

Appropriate planning would provide a variety of units at local level, with training adjusted to individual needs, so that the painfully acquired skills, and the knowledge of a home area, would not be lost. The Pengwern experiment has demonstrated the need for a planned progression, and the need for flexibility in the length of time each individual may require to remain in any given unit. Community training units, in cooperation with Further and Adult Education, must replace the present system of hospital residence and daily attendance at Training Centres, or of family life that is doomed to end after the death of the parents.

If these training homes were linked to an allocation of council housing, the training and preparation would be recognised as relevant, and families would be better able to face the separation from their mentally handicapped children as they approached adult life. It is no longer right to continue a system which means an inevitable admission to a hospital when parents can no longer cope, especially since the declared policy is to run down such institutions.

Pengwern has proved that after appropriate individual training, their youngsters are equipped to live in the community. In general, however, they return to a family home, to a hostel, or to an institution. It is the responsibility of society to see that the labours of those who patiently achieve so much, with so varied a population of mentally handicapped young people, are not in vain. We must ensure that these young adults do not have too long to wait before proving that they can, to a greater extent than previously thought possible, live their lives in a home of their own, with a little help from friends.

Local communities are more likely to accept mentally handicapped people if they are living and learning in the neighbourhood and sharing to the full in community activities, as is the case in the Pengwern project, than if, as is often the case, they are educated in special schools, collected and transported in special buses, spend their adult days in remote training centres and are only rarely encountered in the ordinary social environment.

Planning cannot stop at removing people from hospital into hostels and training homes. The special needs of those young people still at school should be planned for now, and must include preparation for life in a home of their own.

PART THREE

Providing the Homes – Local Authority and
Society Projects

1 Assessing the Problems

The White Paper *Better Services for the Mentally Handicapped*, 1971, proposed that services for mentally handicapped people should be provided within the community, and that the large subnormality hospitals should gradually be run down.

The consultative document of 1981, *Care in the Community*, states that about one third of mentally handicapped people at present in hospital, 15,000 in number, could move out into the community if places were provided. The White Paper also made some predictions of the costs involved, and proposed transferring financial resources from the NHS to local authorities. It is assumed in the 1981 study that the annual cost of care in hospital is approximately £6,000 per patient, and in community residences approximately £2,500.

The report warns that these figures are only to be used as guidelines, noting that, in statistical terms, the per capita cost of hospital patients would rise if their numbers were reduced. The fallacy of comparing services in this way is evident after further examination.

For example, the per capita cost will certainly rise if the cost of the establishment as a whole remains the same. If a 2,000-bed unit is occupied by only 200 persons, but the buildings, heating, lighting and above all staff, are maintained at the same levels, no funds can be made available for transfer to the community.

To plan for the housing of the estimated 15,000 mentally handicapped people within the community pre-supposes the acquisition of suitable homes for them; to find 4,000 or so houses throughout the country, each capable of providing accommodation for a group of four handicapped people and possibly two helpers, does not appear, at first glance, to be an insuperable problem, but it takes no account of those mentally handicapped people currently living at home, who must also be provided with homes in the future.

For the past twenty years there has been an increasing number of residential units provided by voluntary and private agencies, many of which are designed to house upwards of forty residents. The costs involved in these establishments have continued to rise in line with the cost of living index, and have been materially affected in the past ten years by such factors as increased staff salaries, rising maintenance costs and particularly the huge rise in the cost of heating.

The trend to wholesale discharge of patients from hospital, which gained momentum following the publication of the White Paper, was influenced by a general climate of economic optimism. The massive reorganisation of the National Health Service was expected to save money and provide a greatly improved service. Ten years later, however, we can see that neither objective has been achieved, and the steady recession has made a reappraisal of the situation regarding community provision one of urgent concern.

Large units of between twenty and eighty places cannot provide a homely environment, and contrary to expectations, do not provide it cheaply. Such establishments require a high ratio of that most expensive commodity, staff.

Small houses, providing a home for upwards of ten residents, but more usually for three or four people, without resident staff, can be unobtrusively supervised by one or two social workers who can give support to a number of such units without being resident themselves. If these houses and flats are provided by local authorities from their normal housing stock, or by housing associations, these groups of mentally handicapped people are likely to become very desirable tenants. They pay their bills regularly, do not withhold rents and, with the aid of minimum support, maintain their homes in good condition; in short they require much less assistance from the local authority services than many 'problem families' with long-term support needs.

Many local authorities have seized the opportunities provided by the *Consultative Document on Moving Resources for Care in England* to transfer funds from hospital and health allocations to community projects for mentally handicapped people. Some have residential accommodation already, in hostels which have a long waiting list, and must decide what they will provide for those for whom no hostel places exist.

If the hostel is regarded as a training unit or half-way solution, the problem of the best solution for future years is evident.

Young adults, of all levels of ability, often live in hostels when they commence their working lives and leave home for the first time. They neither expect, nor accept, that they will live in a hostel for the rest of their lives, and many of them, within a year, set up in shared flats with friends, once again in a situation which is never contemplated as a home for life.

These stages of preparation for an independent home of their own have not yet been universally accepted as applicable to mentally handicapped people. Too often, a situation designed for one purpose at one stage in life becomes a permanent one, in default of plans for the next stage. There is a strong possibility that the larger hostels will become an outdated institution, with ever increasing problems as the residents and the property age.

The way in which some forward looking local authorities are tackling these problems is demonstrated by projects in widely different areas of the country. A few of them are discussed in the following chapters.

2 Council-Owned Housing

The Chester Road Project – Hereford and Worcester
The population of this authority is 630,000 people, of whom 1,812 are registered as mentally handicapped with the Social Services Departments of the nine local authorities within the county.

By courtesy of Ian Page, social work consultant, mental health, I was able to make an appraisal of the Wyre Forest district provision and to visit Kidderminster in order to examine the amenities provided.

In the conclusion to a consultative report on the general situation within the county, the following statement was made:

> Local people concerned with mental handicap services are typically having to struggle with conflicting pressures and ambiguities in the effort to establish patterns of provision. The economic climate of the early 1980s shows every sign of being distinctly hostile to furthering these efforts.
>
> Comprehensive community based services are the best way of using scarce resources most effectively to meet the special needs of mentally handicapped people. In the longer term, not only is their contribution increased, but there will be a reduction in expenditure on expensive hospital places for people. who basically need care, support and further education and training, rather than medical services.

In the Wyre Forest area the group homes and hostels which serve those attending the adult training centre are full and have waiting lists, as does the training centre, but in Kidderminster ten mentally handicapped people now live as council tenants in ordinary estates, following preparation at a small house in Chester Road.

The scheme was initiated in 1977 and was made possible by an offer from the County Council to the Social Services Department of the Local Authority. Originally intended as a hostel, or a half-way house, for groups of men and women due for discharge from mental handicap hospitals, the Chester Road Centre has successfully prepared long-stay hospital residents for independent living, largely as a result of the initiative of the officer in charge and her staff, none of whom are resident.

There are places for eight mentally handicapped people, and the staff includes a full-time residential social worker, two part-time social work assistants who give twenty hours each per week, and a peripatetic staff member who assists at the structured training sessions.

The house is an ordinary semi-detached late Victorian house, on a main road and no different from its neighbours. There are double bedrooms, all on one floor, with a larger than usual bathroom, previously converted from a bedroom, and a small attic room which serves as a modest office. The ground floor has two reception rooms and a reasonably sized kitchen with the bare essentials of a large family home, a small laundry in an outhouse and drying facilities.

The small staff not only instruct the residents in the basic skills of using a telephone, shopping, reading and writing, but achieve a high standard of cookery and laundry in far from ideal conditions. The results of their efforts in these two fields were apparent on the day I visited Chester Road itself, and endorsed later in the private houses to which the early residents had moved. One man in particular, living in a shared flat, provided for tea a sponge cake cooked by himself, and was wearing a perfectly laundered and ironed shirt – his own work. He volunteered the information that he had benefited by the teaching he had received from the officer in charge at Chester Road, and told me of an occasion when he had visited her in her own home: he had found her ironing her husband's pyjamas and had asked why she had not extended instruction in laundry work to him.

This particular resident was in a flat belonging to a housing association which he shared with another mentally handicapped man who was in employment. He himself had just been declared redundant, in common with hundreds of people in the area, badly hit by the collapse of local industry, particularly the carpet trade. He had an interview in the next few days for work with a major retail food chain, and asked me if I thought the suit and, in particular, his shirt, would do credit to the occasion. His smart appearance was reflected in the immaculate kitchen and in the general standard of housekeeping in the whole flat.

The residents in Chester Road may be there for two years – the longest stay to date – or for a period as short as three months. Most come from mental handicap hospitals, and many have been inmates for as long as twenty years. I met a woman there, now in her mid-forties, who had been in hospital for over twenty-four years, but now, after only ten months of living in Chester Road, she was already on the local authority housing waiting list.

All the staff support a common philosophy initiated by the officer in charge: a sensitive appreciation of the individual needs of each resident and a personal programme designed to meet these needs. Since the ultimate aim is independence, emphasis is placed on all aspects of self care, and in particular money management and budgeting. These people will eventually have a rent book and be responsible for all outgoings, so they must be instructed in expenditure and saving. All have a building society account and learn to save for larger expenses.

One feature of people who have always lived in staffed institutions is a determination to preserve privacy and a general mistrust of any invasion of this, The social worker who explained the training to me said that one man was most suspicious of the deductions made from his statutory benefits during his preliminary training at the hostel. He was only convinced when she suggested that the whole amount should be changed into small denomination notes and silver; she then sat down and actually divided the whole into the various small piles for rent, food, toilet requisites, savings and pocket money. At the conclusion he asked where her pile was, and she explained that she did not have a personal share, since the social services paid her a salary. It was with difficulty that he was persuaded not to make an allocation to the staff from his own pocket money, and he was no longer worried that any deductions were unfair. It is this kind of

LIFE IN HOSPITAL

Joseph John Deacon
lived in St. Lawrence's
Hospital, Caterham, from
the age of seven until he
moved into a purpose-built
bungalow in his fifty-
eighth year.

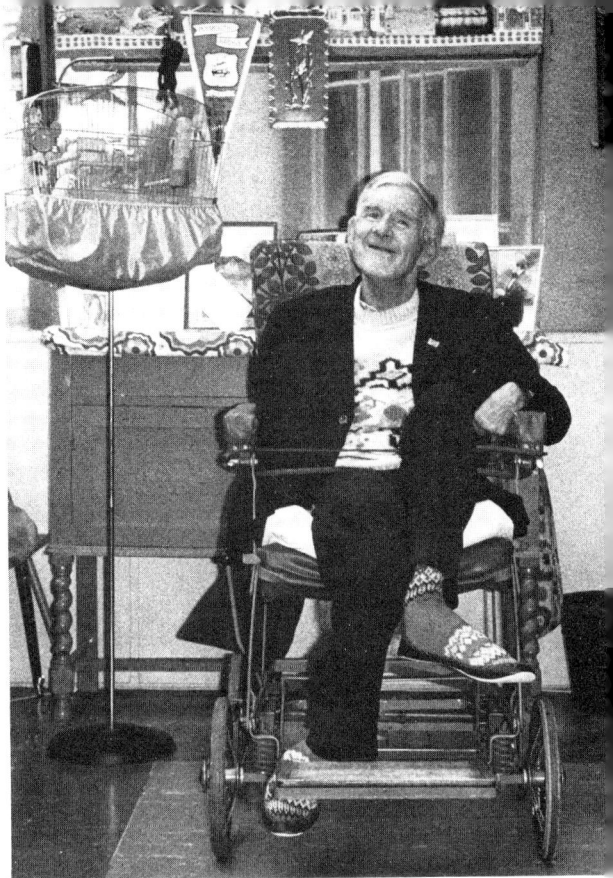

In a corner of the
verandah, he created a
small personal refuge and
received many friends as a
result of his book *Tongue
Tied*.

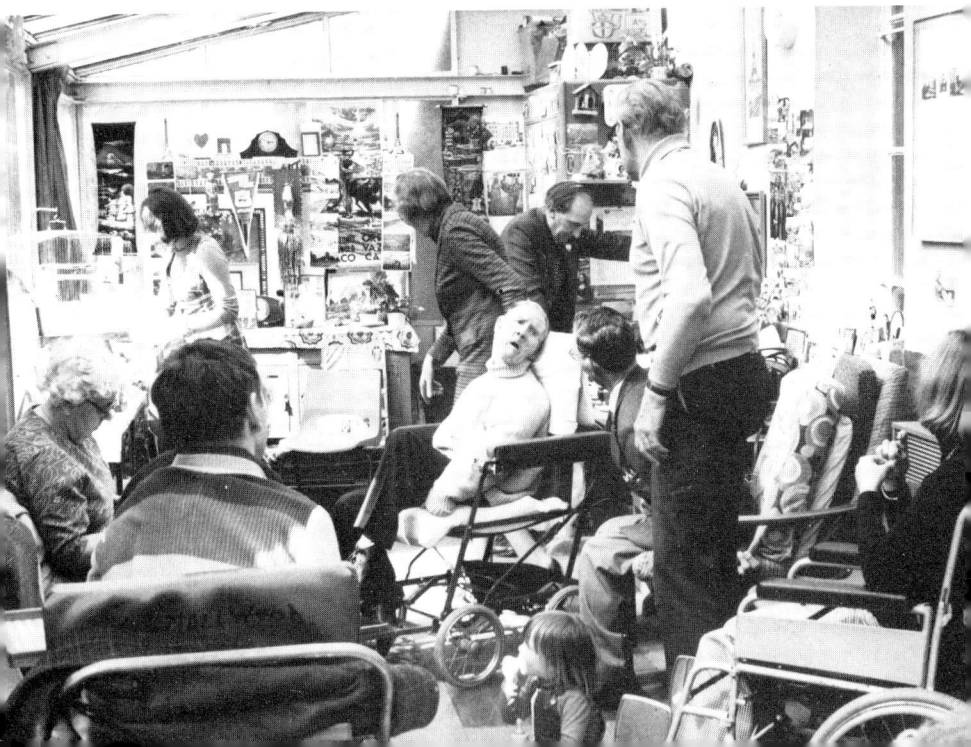

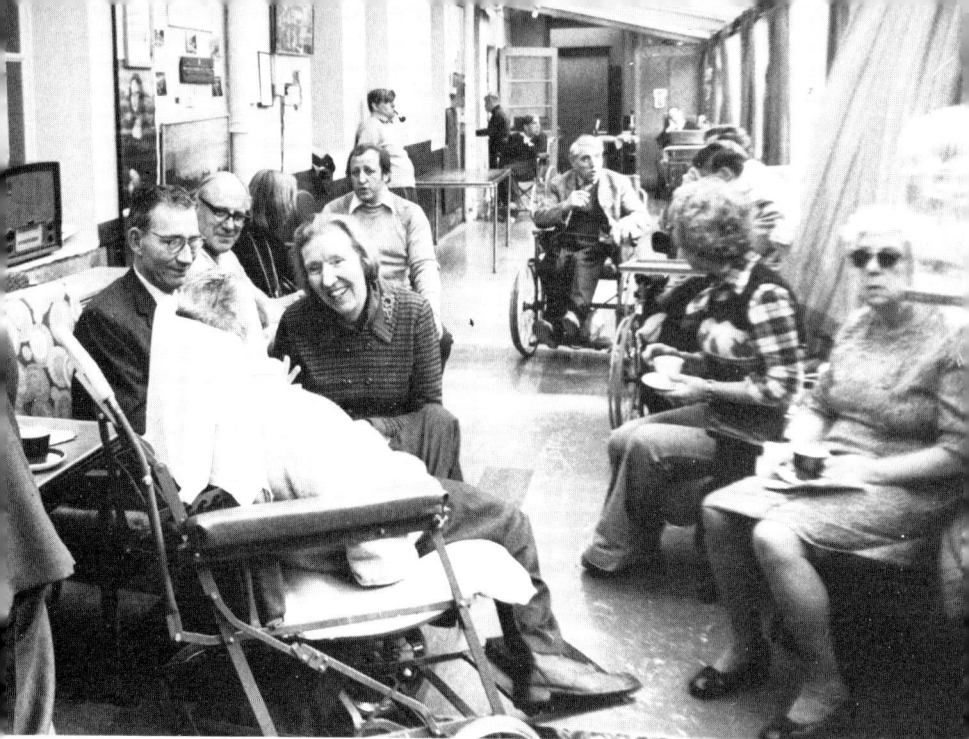

There is little privacy in the long corridors and wards, but the four friends
were able to get about in the hospital grounds.

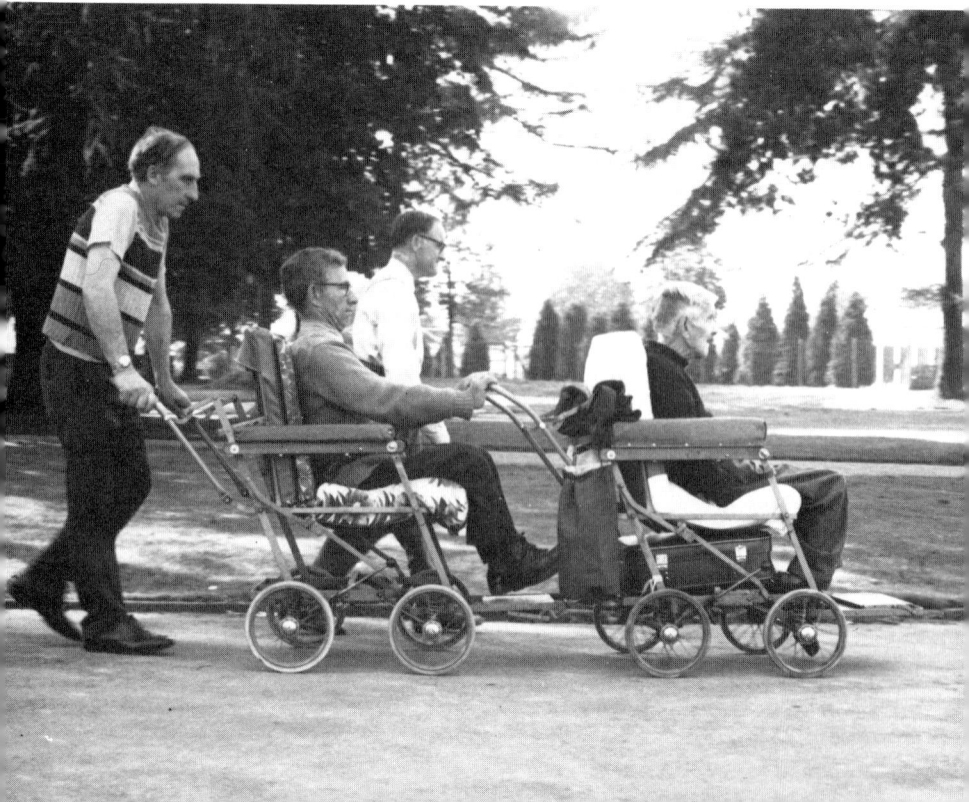

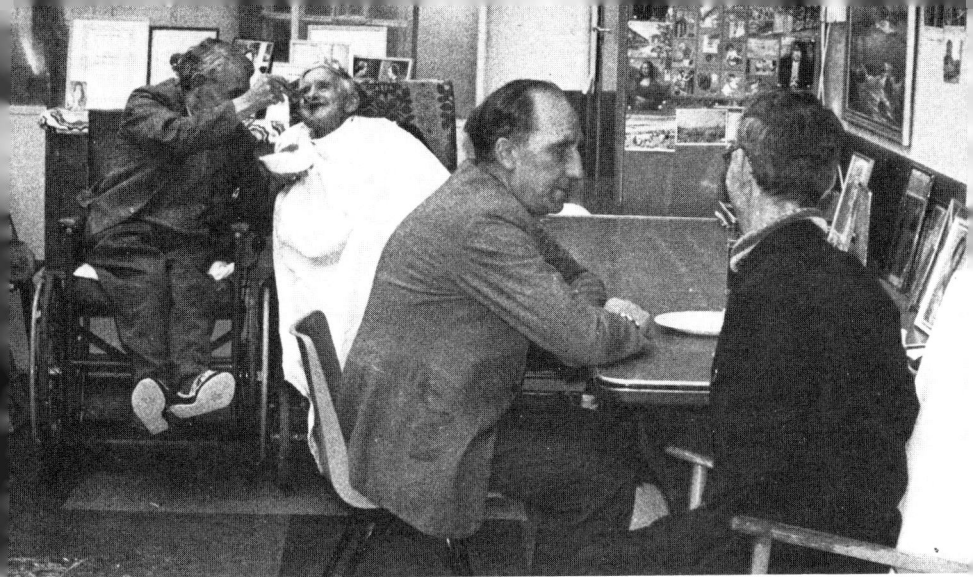

Patients help each
other in hospitals of
this kind; Joey could
do nothing for himself,
but with the help of
friends he wrote his
life story.

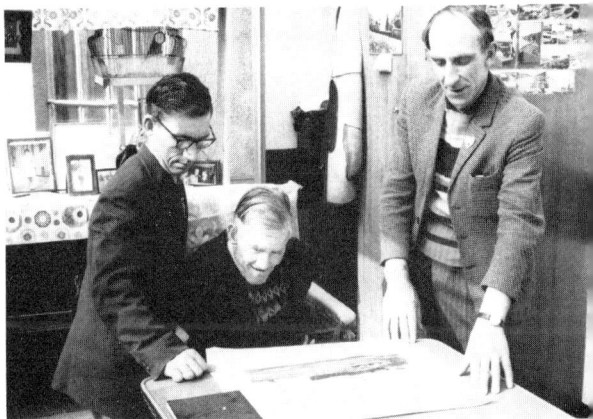

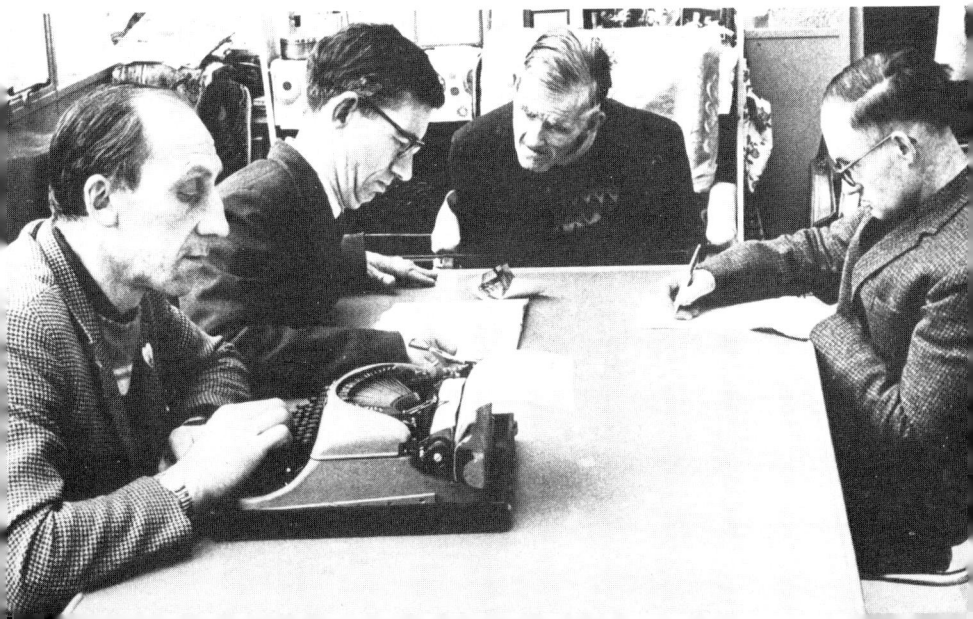

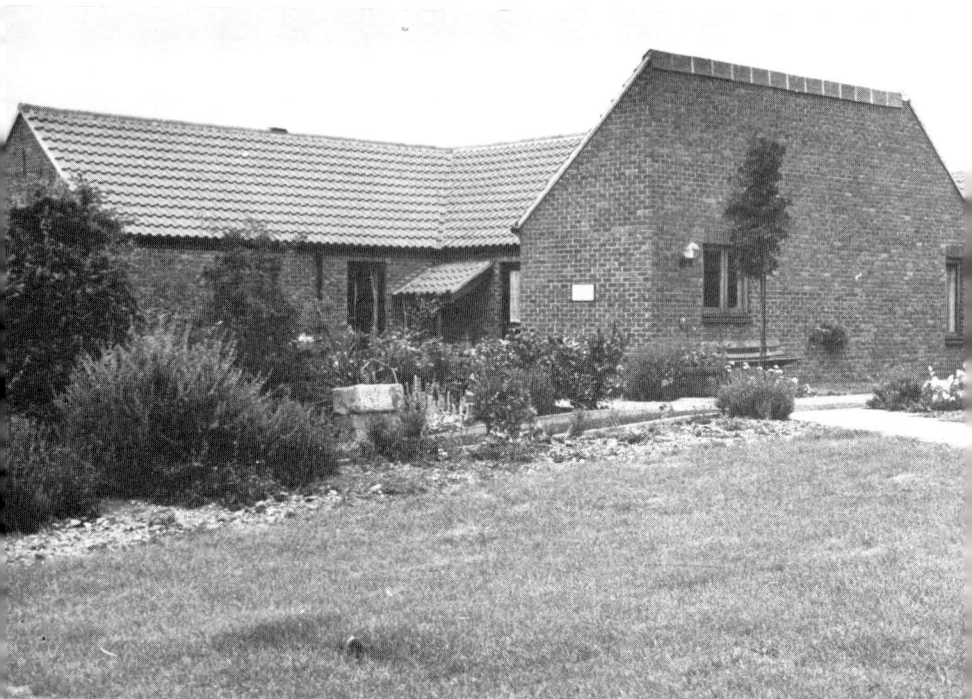

The purpose-built bungalow, Amsterdam, was opened in 1977. Joey moved in, with the framed editions of translations of his book.

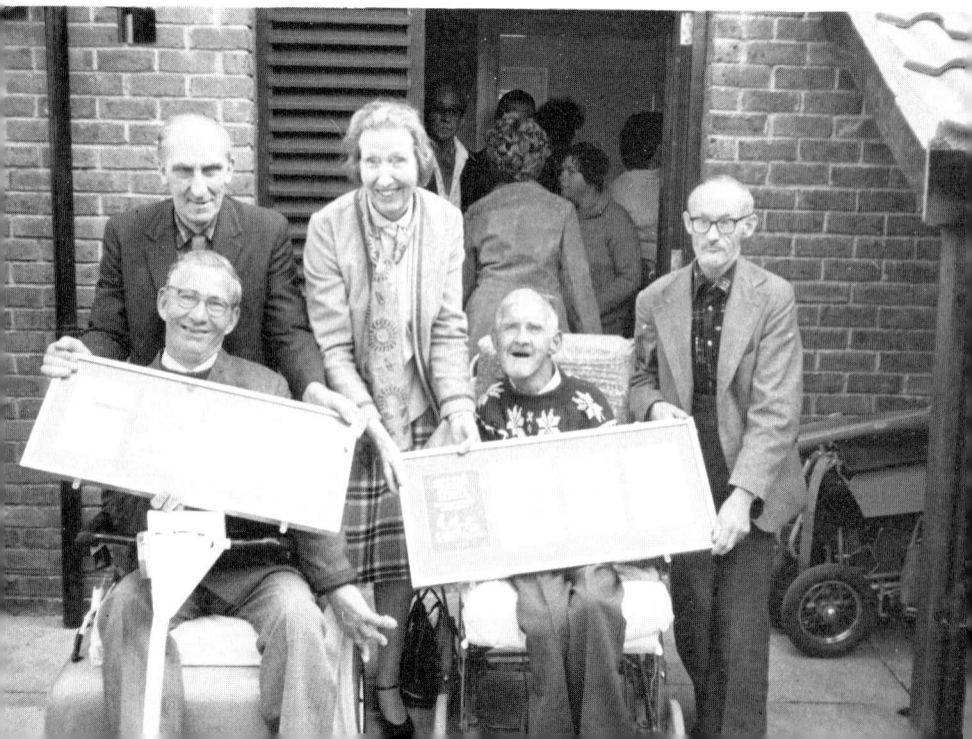

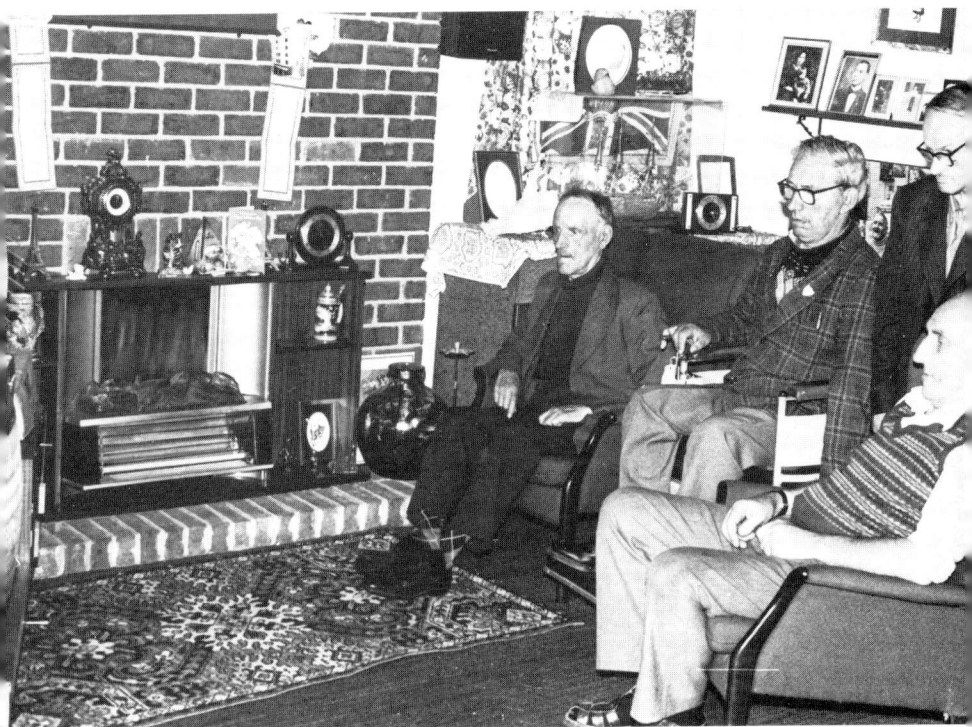

They enjoy today an ordinary life, with ordinary pleasures, and share the chores of shopping and cooking for themselves.

Photographs on pages 1–5 by permission of St. Lawrence's Hospital, Caterham

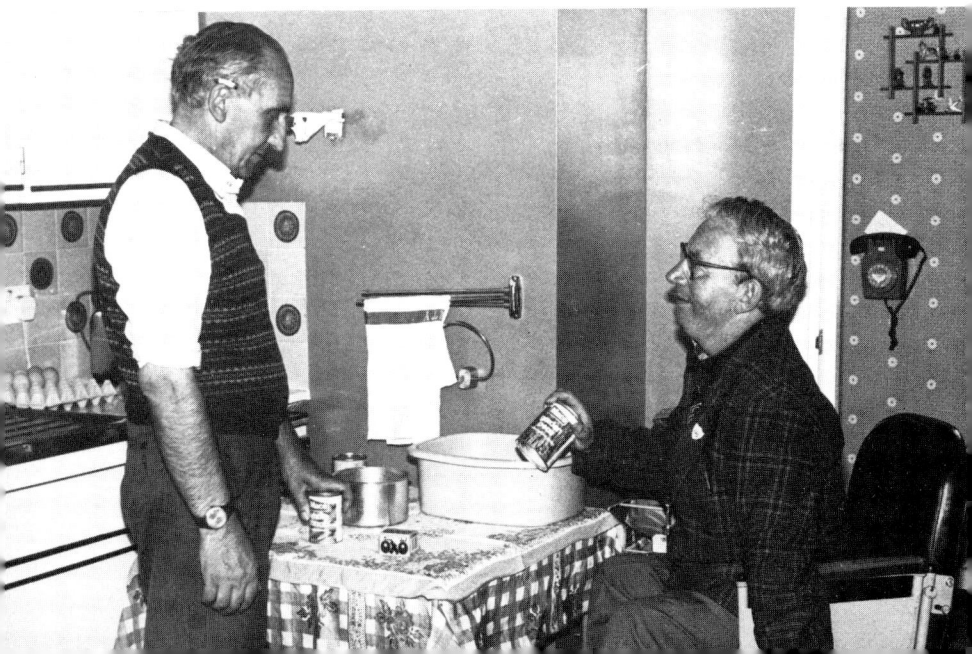

THE PENGWERN HALL PROJECT

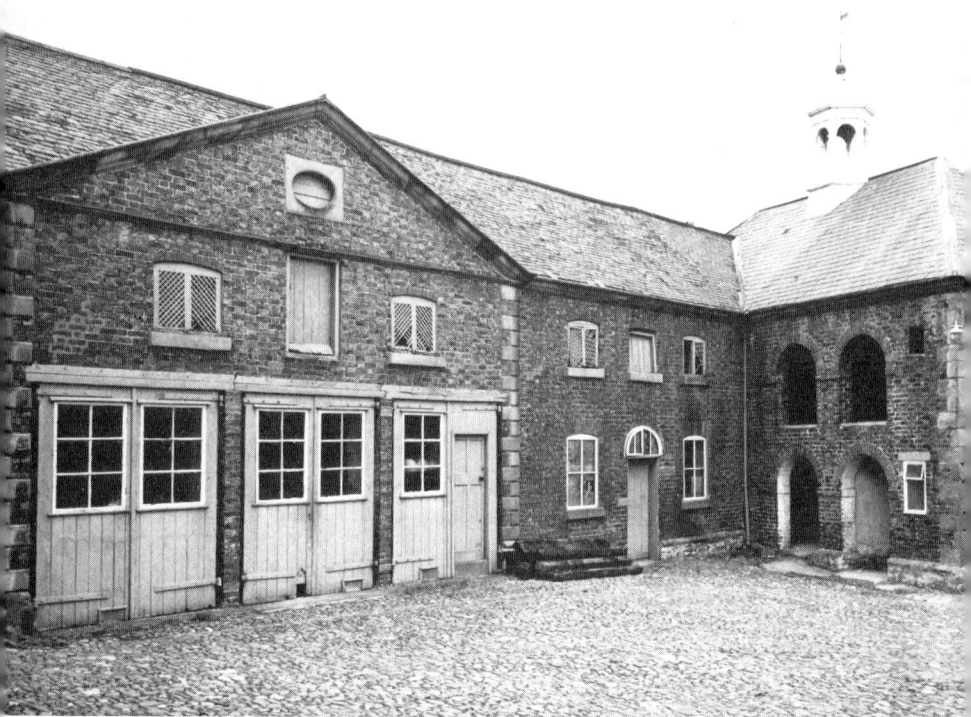

This derelict annexe sparked off the Pengwern project of preparing young people to live independently. They worked on all aspects of the conversion, under skilled supervision.

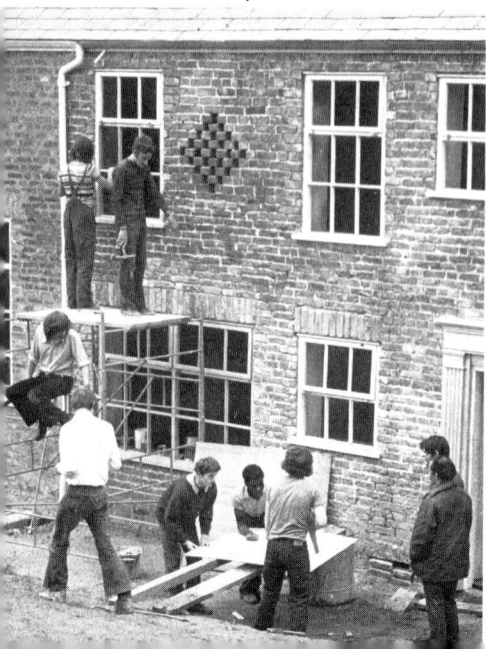

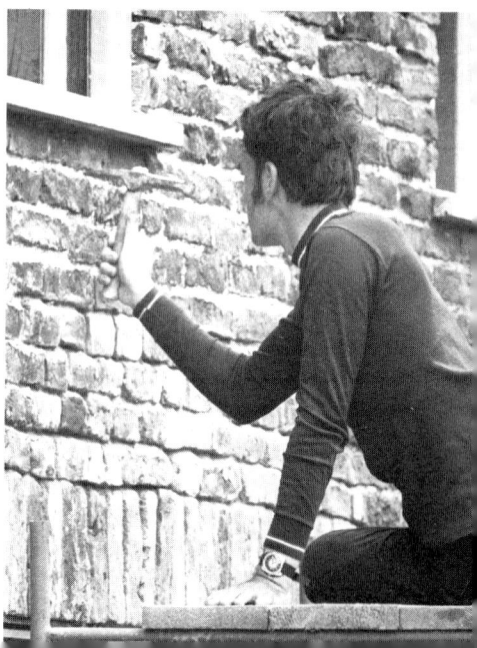

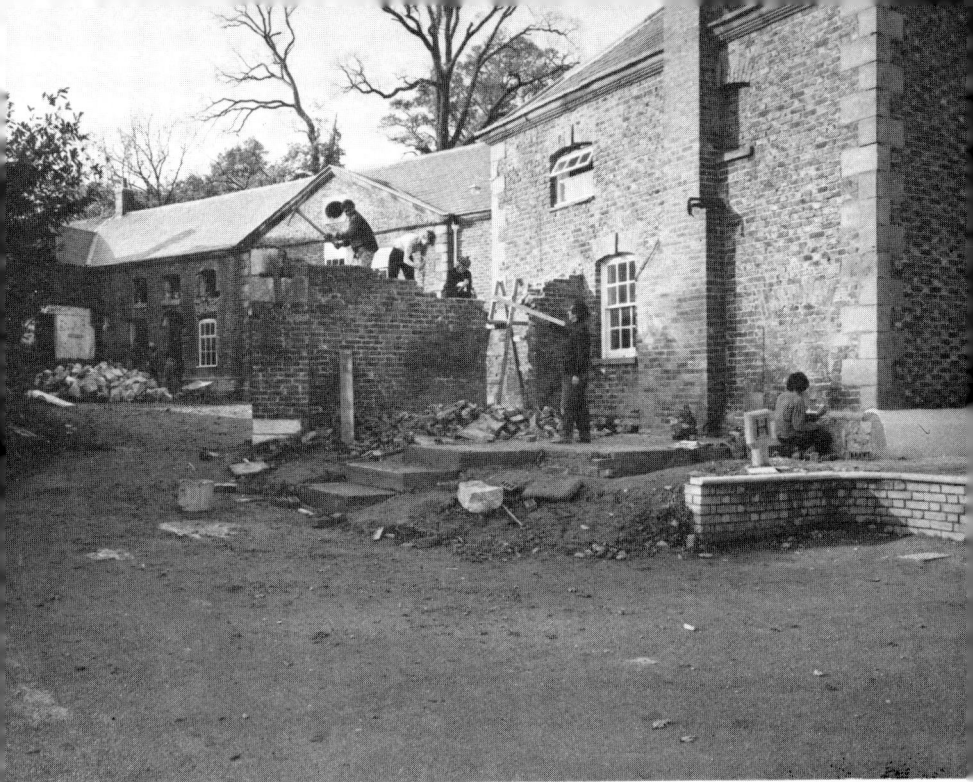

The finished improvement, which provides units of self-contained accommodation in the old stable block at the rear.

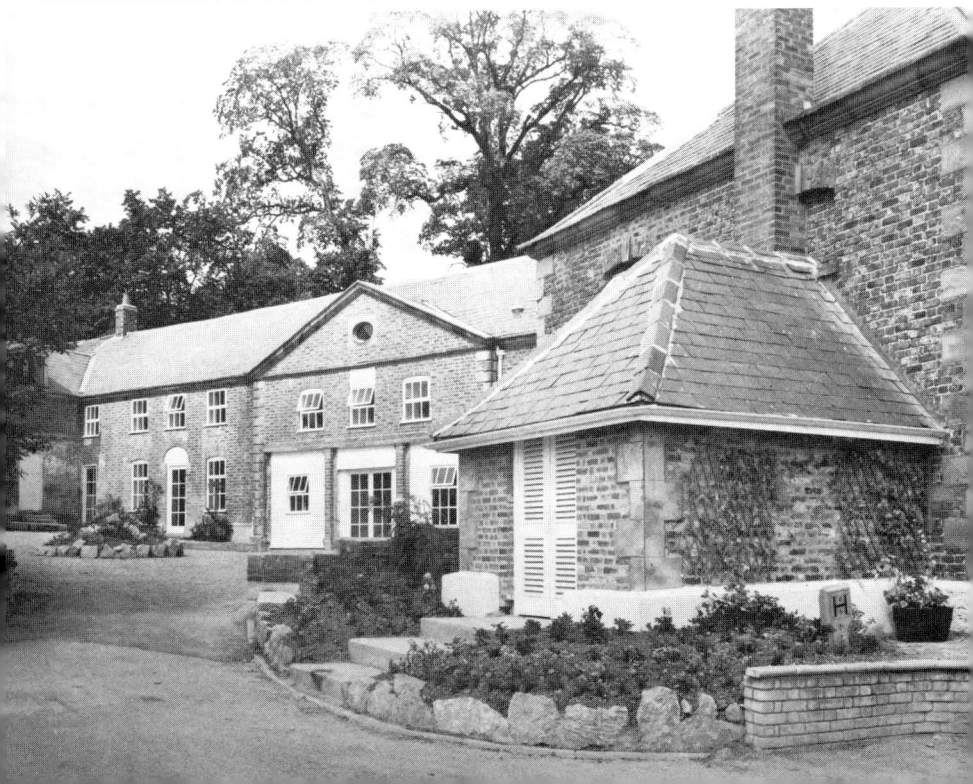

LEARNING TO COPE

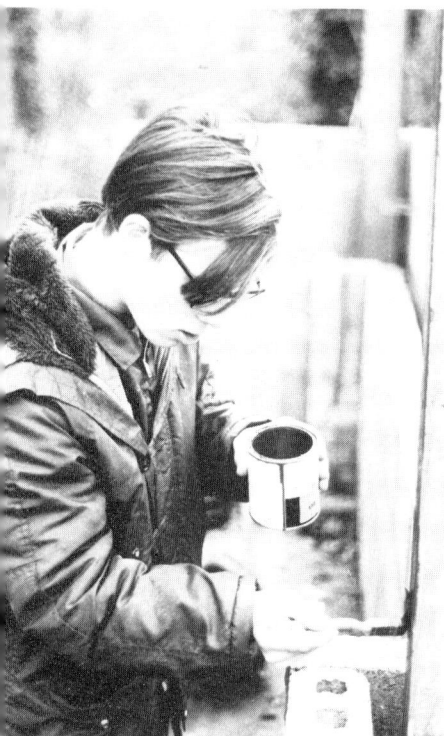

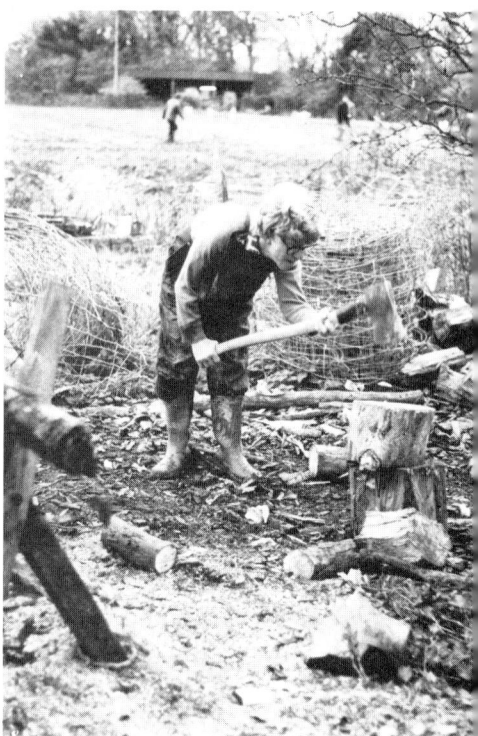

All the do-it-yourself skills are taught, and the young people learn to use powered equipment as well as hand tools.

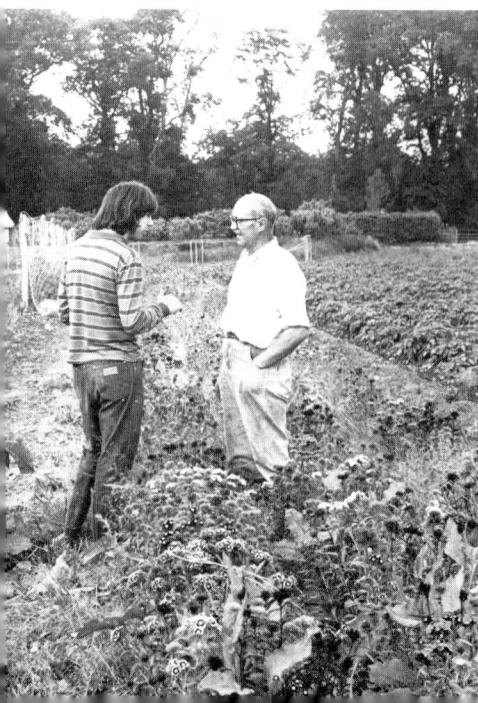

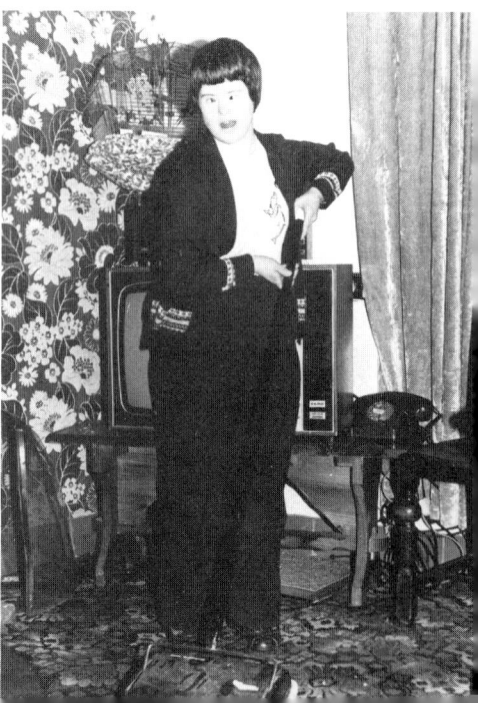

FROM SHOPPERS TO SHOPKEEPERS

From learning how to plan for meals and budget for shopping, young trainees now run their own village stores.

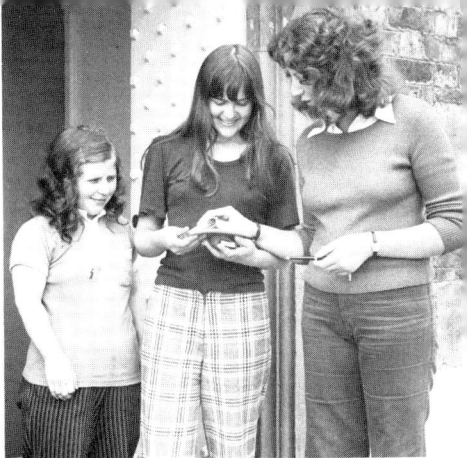

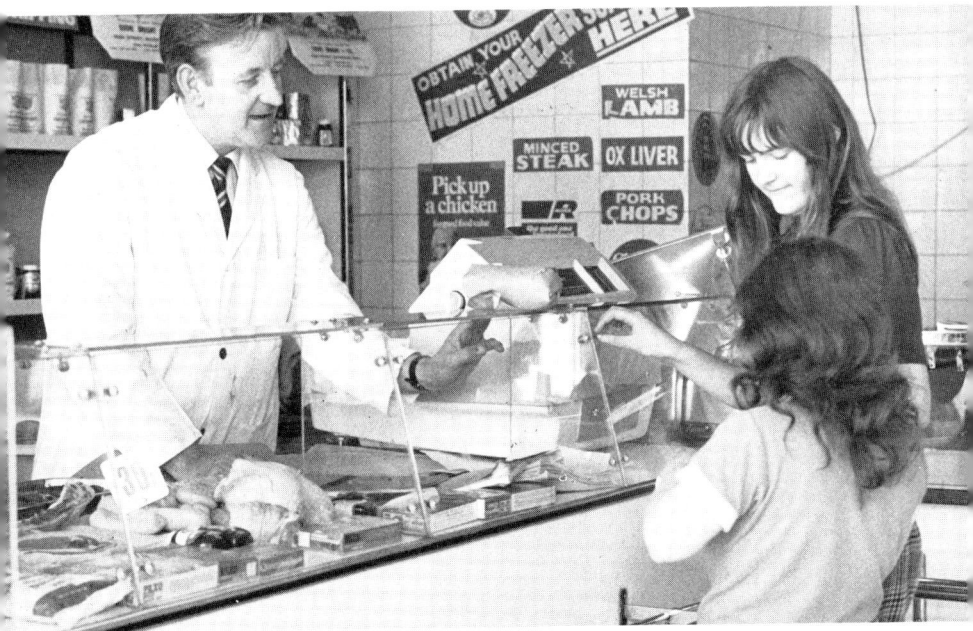

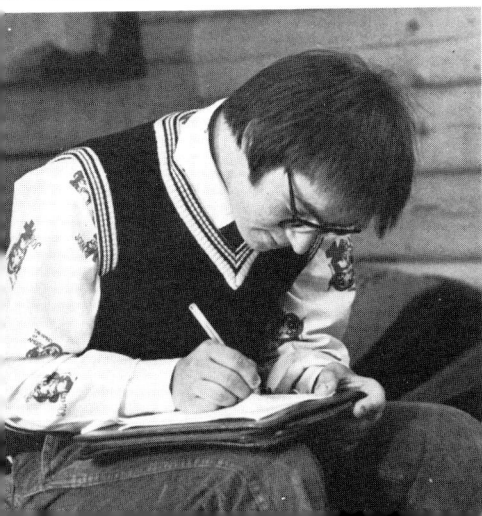

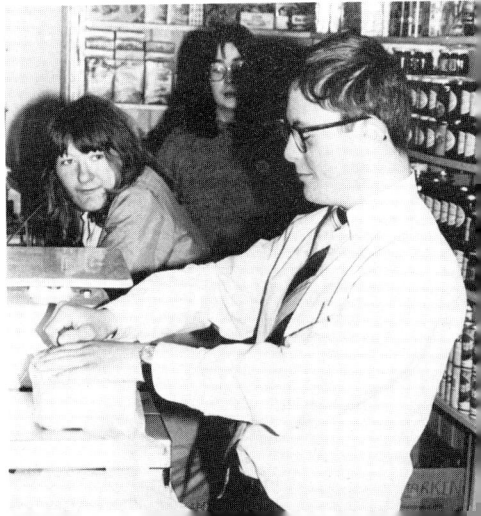

RESTORING A HOUSE

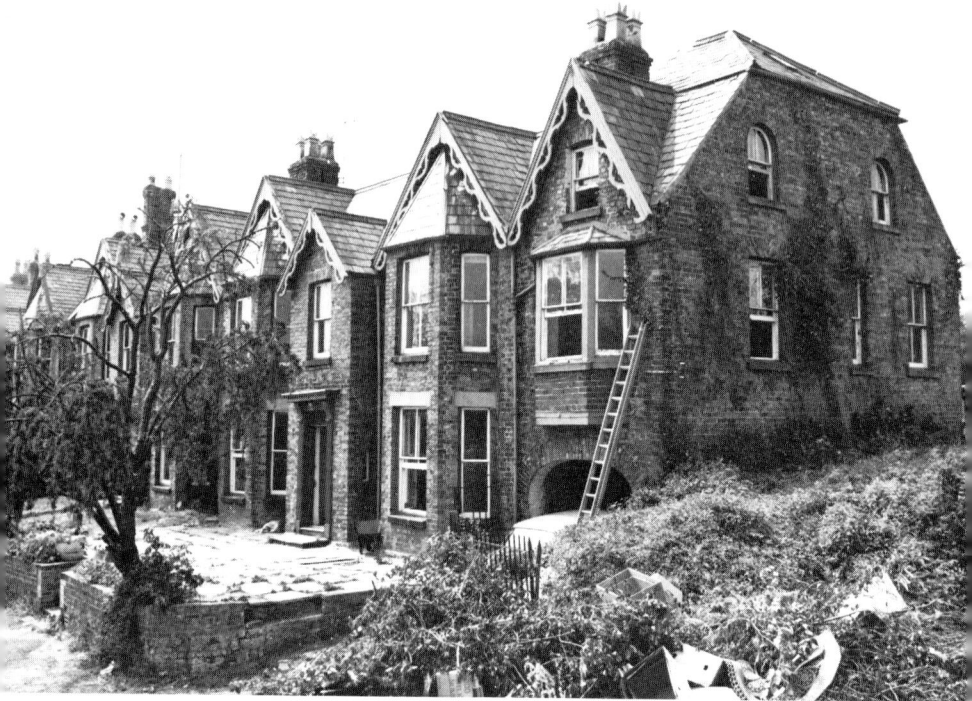

The next stage is restoring a house in the community, using the experience gained at Pengwern Hall.

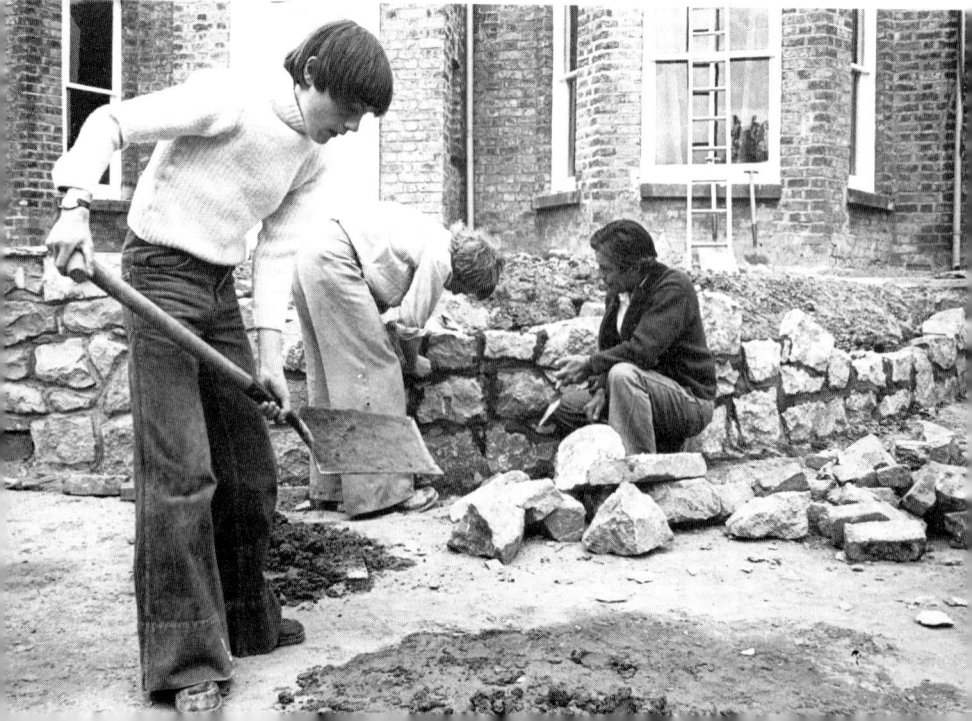

TO A HOME

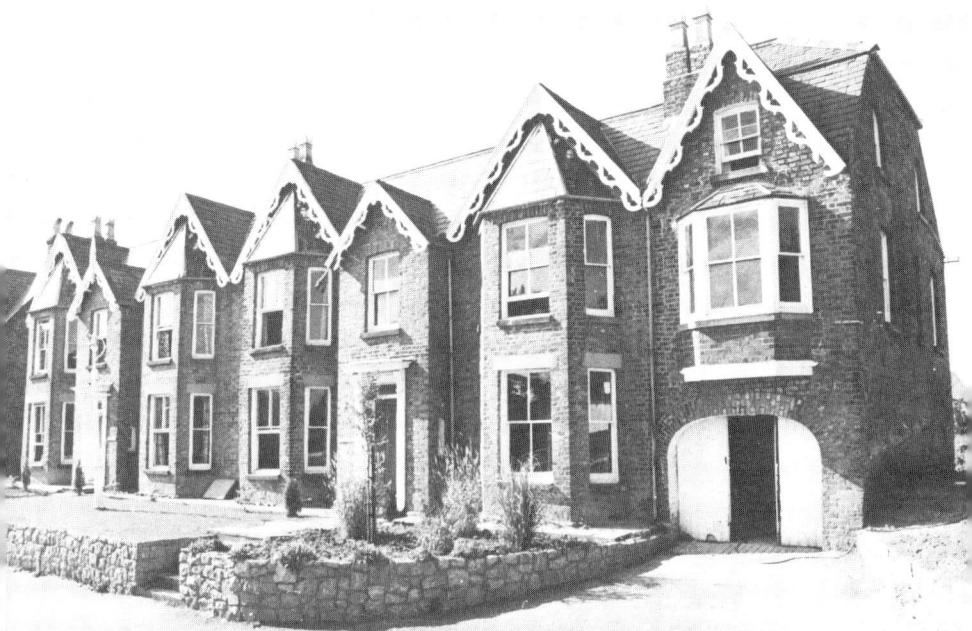

'The house' becomes 'our house' and the resident family welcome visitors.

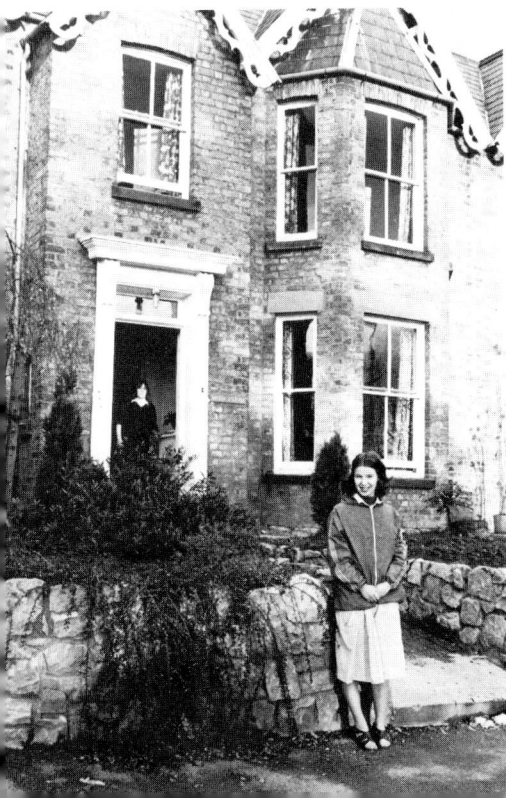

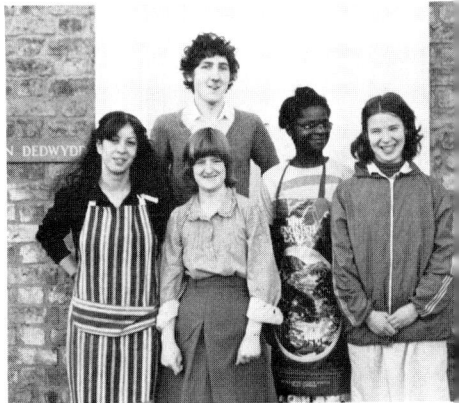

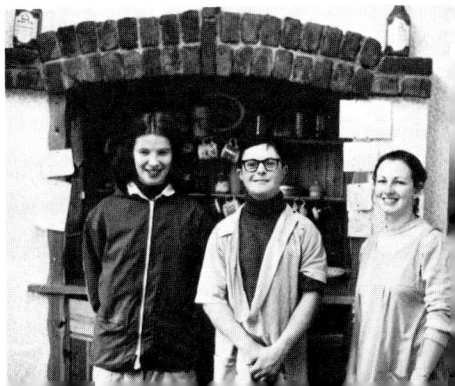

A COUNTRY COTTAGE

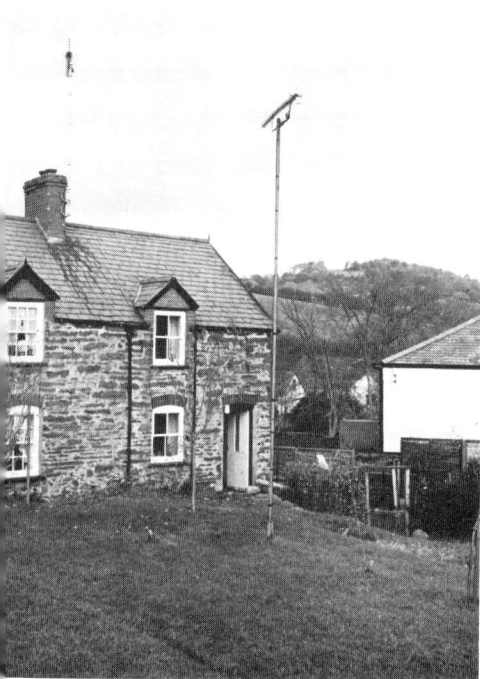

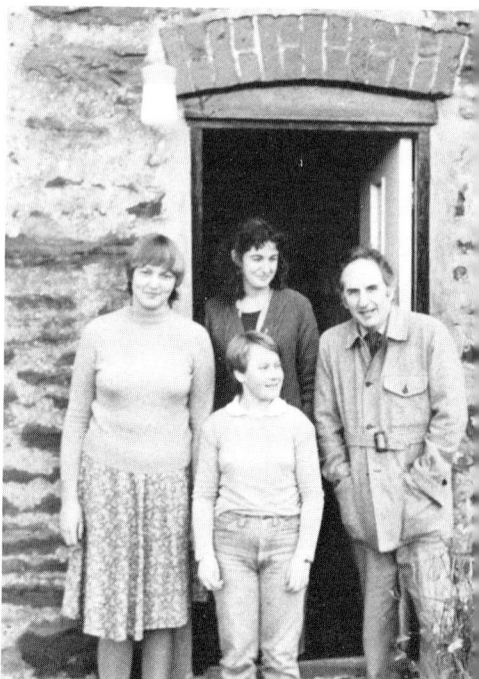

Next, a country cottage accommodates youngsters who now live some distance from Pengwern, but are closely in touch with the Director, Martin Weinberg.

Photographs on pages 6–12 by permission of Pengwern Hall, Rhuddlan

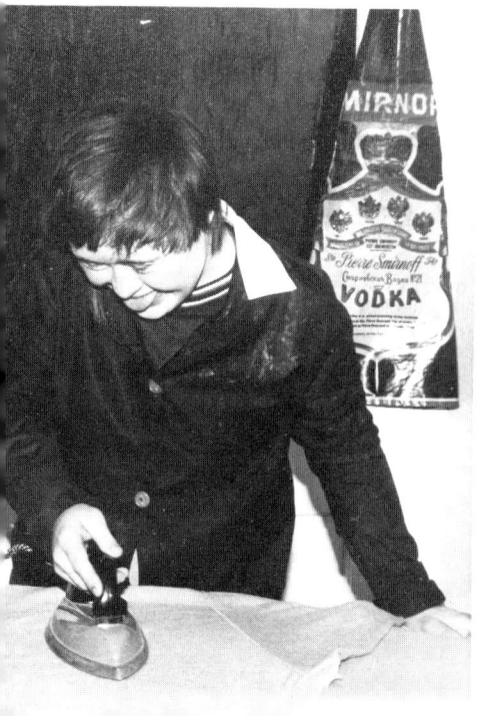

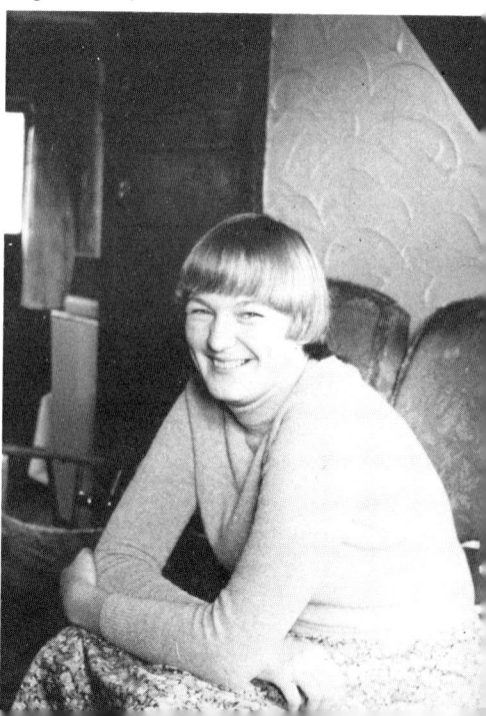

ORDINARY HOUSES IN A LONDON BOROUGH

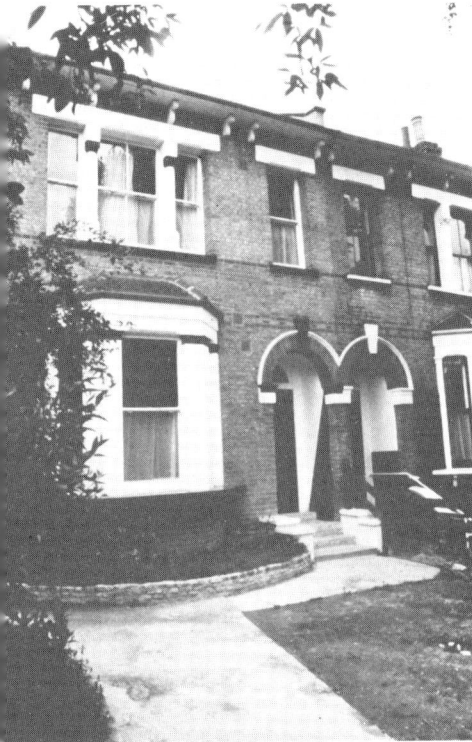

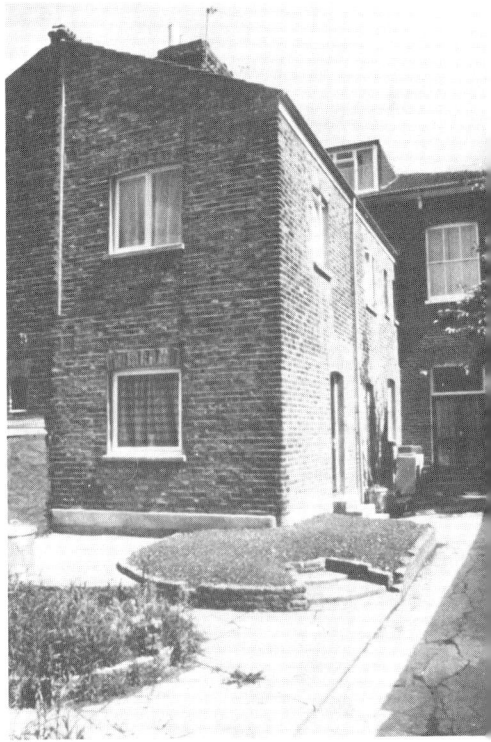

Typical small suburban properties can provide homes for people now living in hospital.

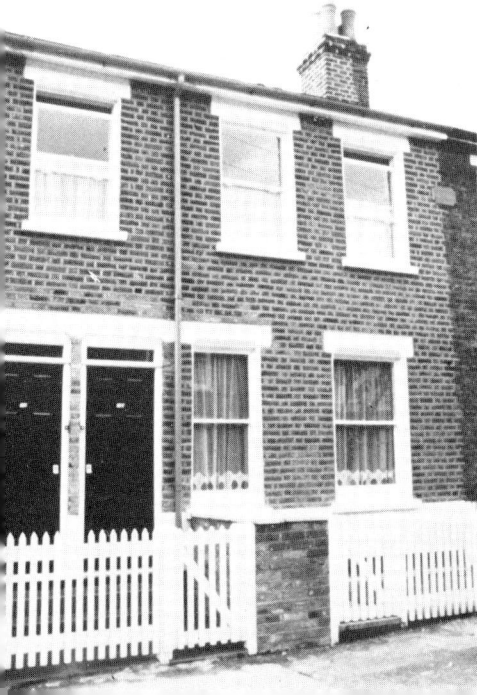

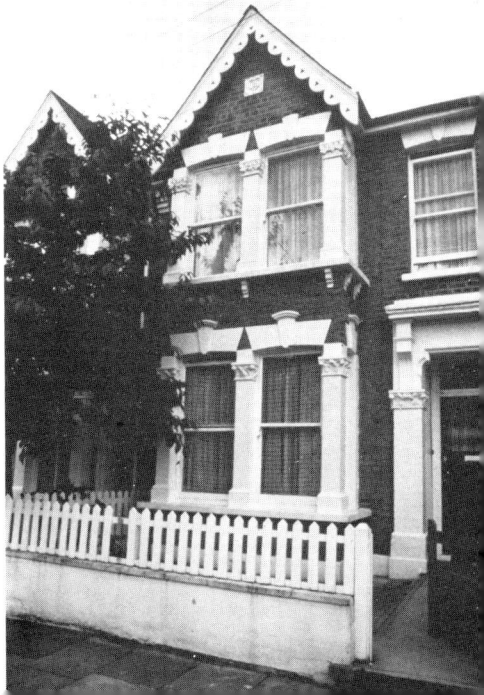

MODERN FLATS PROVIDE HOMES

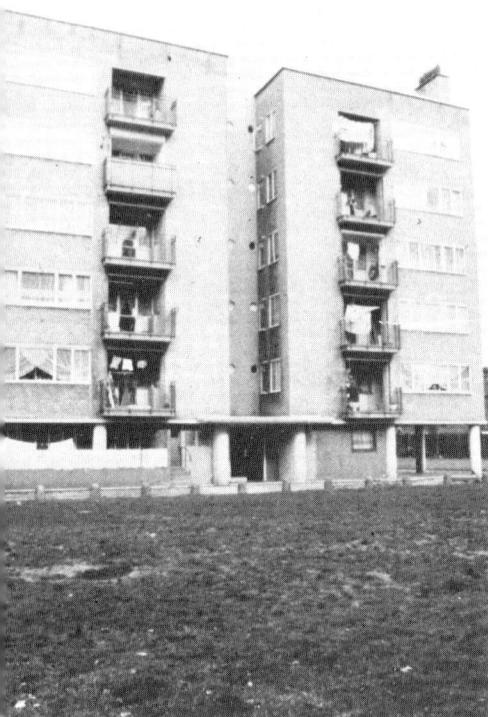

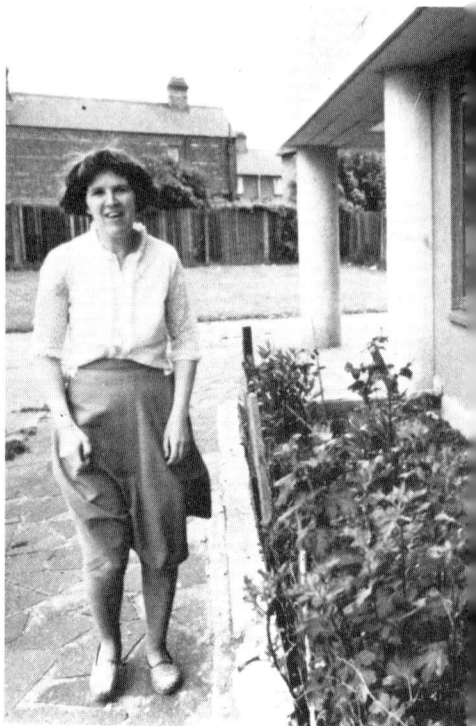

Modern high rise flats have made it possible for others.

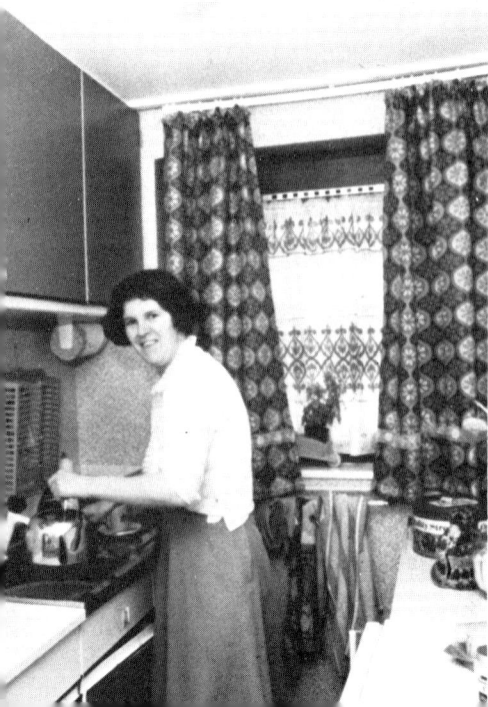

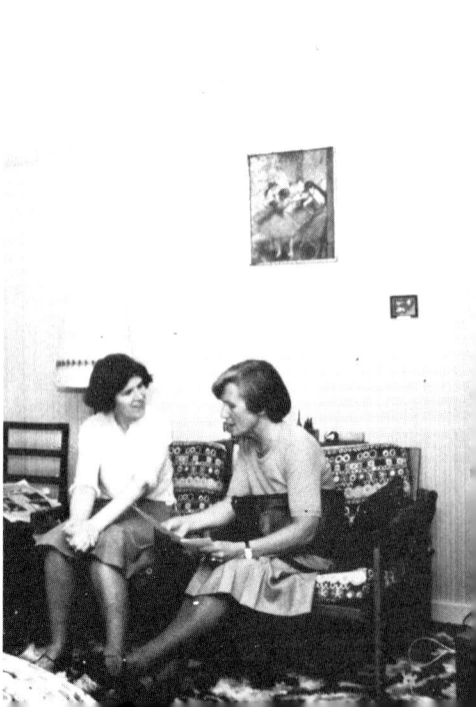

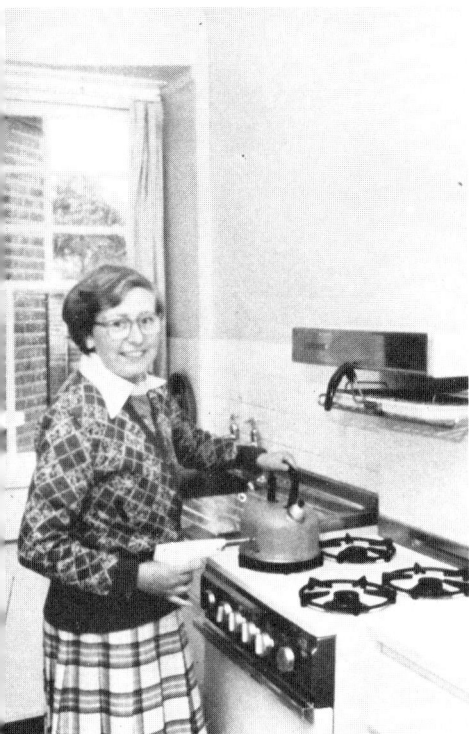

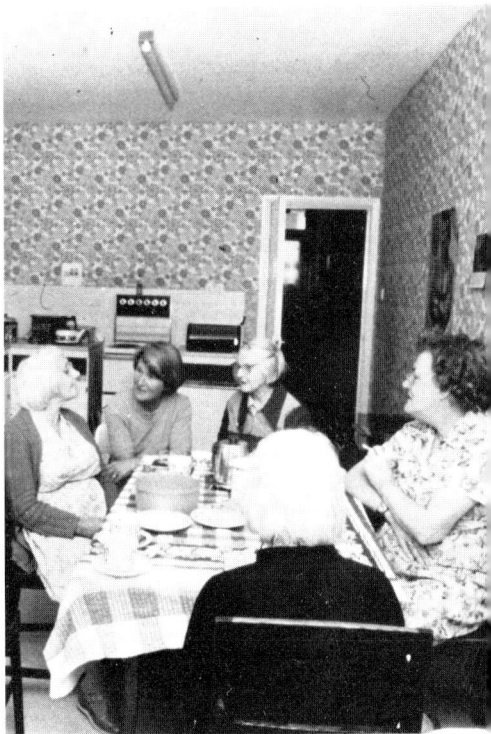

After training and living as a group, some prefer to live alone, with a pet for company.

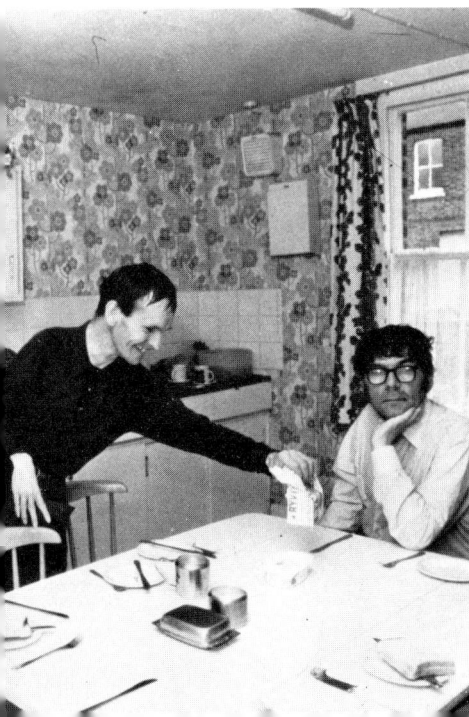

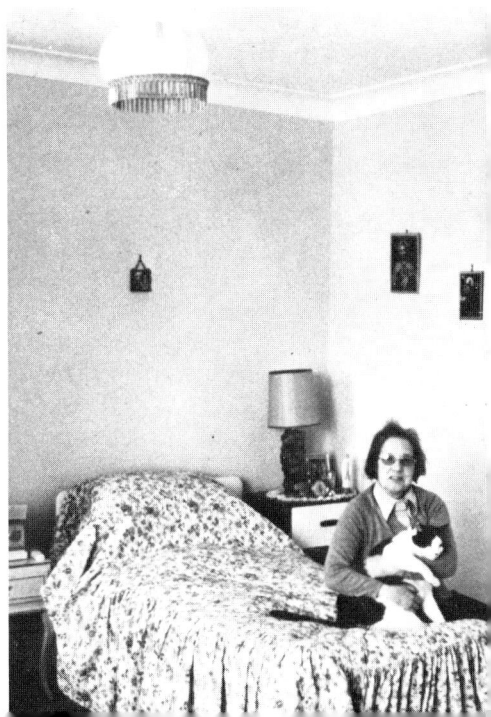

LIKE OTHER PEOPLE

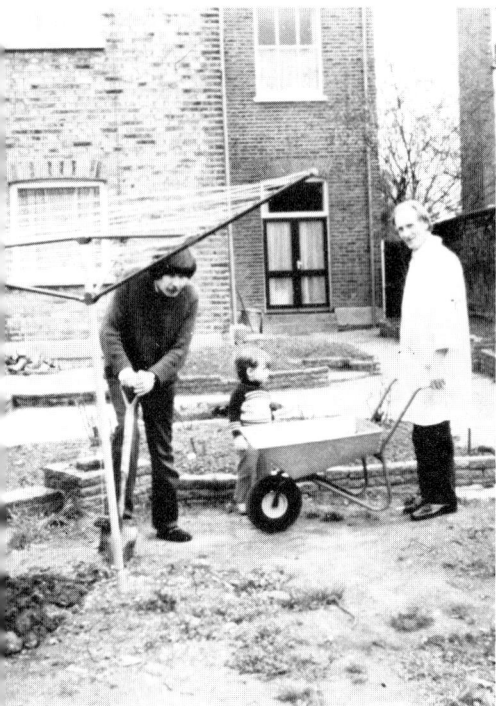

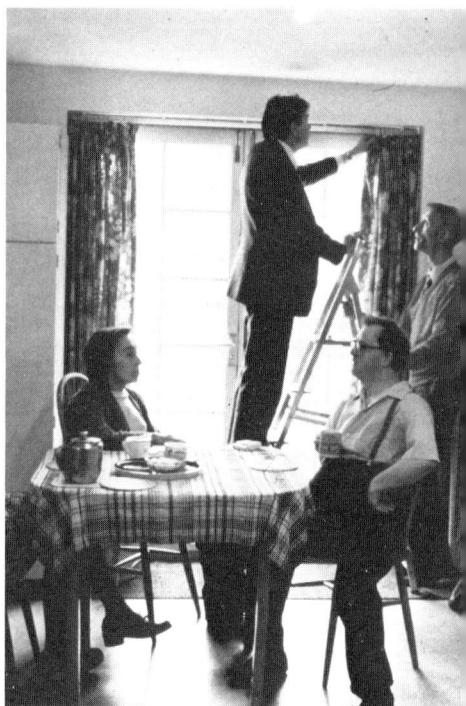

Whether living as a group or alone, all continue to receive help and support for the adventure of living in the community.

Photographs on pages 13–16 by permission of Alex Sowerby

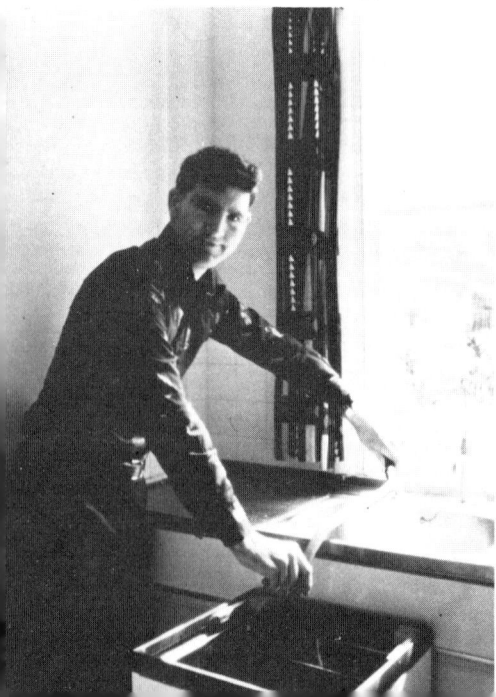

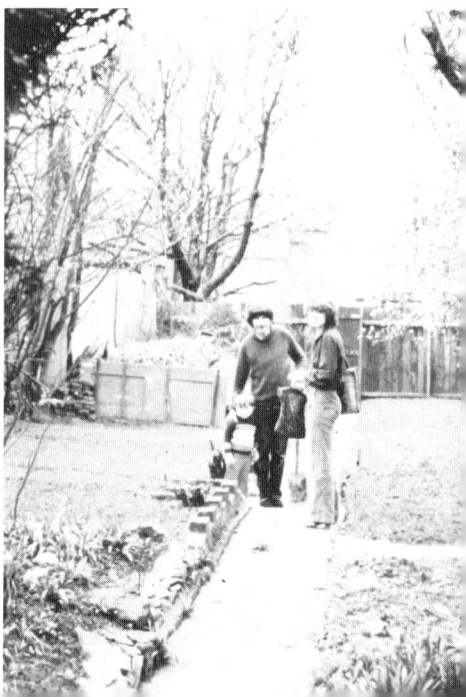

imaginative, practical and patient instruction that enables the move from the Chester Road Centre to be successfully made, in almost every case.

One of the few failures has been with a resident in her mid-twenties, admitted from her family home. The parents were anxious that she should learn to live independently, but she was unable to achieve the break from her parents' home, in spite of two periods of instruction. Not everyone in the ordinary population is temperamentally suited to independence, and mentally handicapped people have as diverse personalities as others.

The instruction at Chester Road is divided between two or three regular instruction periods in cooking and catering, hygiene and sex education, literacy and numeracy, as well as the daily practical skills of running the home: cleaning, rubbish disposal, use of the washing machine and gardening.

All members of the Chester Road team have a warm and caring attitude towards their residents. The weekly cookery class is much enjoyed and evidence of the very high level of practical skill of the staff member who instructs. She is not a qualified caterer or domestic science teacher, but a thoroughly experienced housewife used to managing with ordinary, often less than ideal equipment, and it is these skills which she has passed on to her students. Each of the private houses I visited subsequently had kitchen provision vastly superior to that in Chester Road, but in each house I was offered refreshments, which bore witness to the efficiency of the instruction received. The Chester Road Centre is proof of the advantages of accepting what is offered and of improvisation by dedicated people, rather than a policy of waiting for the ideal situation to be provided.

The staff keep a 'Communications' book in which each member records his or her personal work with each resident, and includes observations of particular difficulties. This is in no sense an official record, but supplements the returns required by the Social Services Department. All agreed that these records and comments were an invaluable help when special difficulties and crises arose.

At the end of the first two years a request was made by the officer in charge for four residents to be placed on the council waiting list for houses. The initial approach required much hard argument, and the allocation was only made subject to continued supervision by the Chester Road staff.

Once the first allocation was made, a subsequent allocation of a two-place flat in a housing association project was requested. It was common practice for prospective tenants to be approved by others and an adverse reaction was received, some existing tenants going so far as to petition against the two mentally handicapped men. The warden of the block, however, was in favour, and determined backing from Chester Road carried the day. After more than a year, and one change of resident when one of the original tenants moved out of the district, the other tenants accept the situation and have made friends with the two men; they are prime favourites of the warden, giving less trouble than others, rather than more.

As I have indicated above, the high standard of equipment and maintenance in this flat is a tribute to the emphasis on saving and budgeting – furnishings and carpets were bought by the men, both employed at the time of occupation, with cash from savings. The Chester Road training does not endorse hire purchase; the principle is to save first until the items can be afforded.

The residents in a three-bedroomed council house were equally comfortably installed. Here there were two men and two women. Both the women were in local domestic employment, and one man attended the training centre. The other man had just been declared redundant and was undertaking more of the domestic management and cooking. I visited them shortly after the worst spell of winter weather experienced in the Midlands for almost twenty years, but the mentally handicapped residents had coped as well as anyone else with the appalling conditions. Their main concern was the size of their gas bill for central heating, and they needed considerable reassurance from the visiting staff member from Chester Road that between four building society accounts there was ample to meet the bills.

This group of four people had been the first to be allocated council housing, and it was obvious that the care in their selection, and the patient supervision, had resulted in their success and the consequent willingness of the Local Authority to consider subsequent allocations. The staff regard the residents, once moved out, as ordinary council tenants, and do not visit unless invited. However, they are obviously regarded as friends, and are on 24-hour telephone availability for advice and practical help.

The residents in this house had been asked if they would like a visitor, and I was most warmly welcomed. They explained that on Saturday mornings they did the weekly shopping, so they had only just finished their domestic chores, but they insisted that I explore the whole house and admire, in particular, a kitten they had just adopted. There were personal belongings and pictures in each bedroom, and the men had a black and white television set in theirs, in addition to the colour set in the sitting-room shared by them all. They were highly articulate, expressing their feelings about living on the estate and their particular pleasure in being opposite the school.

Like any other incoming council tenants, when Chester Road residents are allocated houses, the neighbours are not informed who they are, and each household makes its own contacts with neighbours in accordance with the wishes of both parties. This practice must certainly preclude the misconceptions which so often prejudice community placements from the start.

The last house I visited had only been occupied for one year – the tenants were, in fact, organising a celebration for the next weekend and were inviting some of the current Chester Road residents. This house was more than a mile away from Chester Road, but the tenants, a man and three women, still returned there for a regular weekly meeting, at which current problems and future plans were discussed. At that moment, arrangements were being decided for the summer holiday, which the staff and residents normally take as a group.

There was one younger member in this house who was more outgoing than the others; she described to me some of the problems she had experienced in the past. She said that she had a child, living with her mother, and admitted that she had been very difficult with the staff at Chester Road. 'I once rang up one of them at her home, at two o'clock in the morning, to tell her I was going to leave this house – just walk out – but I didn't go, though I had packed up my things.' Surely an example of dedication – staff who can accept 2 am phone calls!

The regular weekly meetings were a means of letting off steam, of identifying and modifying attitudes. I was told that 'we can say what we like about the staff, and complain if we want. Sometimes I think it is a waste of time, especially in winter when it's dark and we have to walk there and back at night.'

The company on these walks of the one man was appreciated by the three women, one of middle age and two younger. Incidentally, in both houses the relationship between the men and women residents was easy, comparable to that of brothers and sisters in an ordinary household. As far as a casual visitor like myself is concerned, the fears expressed by some people of the dangers inherent in mixed sex accommodation for mentally handicapped people seem likely to be less well-founded than for the ordinary population.

Mentally handicapped people who have lived in institutions and achieved community residence are acutely aware of the need to conform, and are not willing to risk the disapproval of their neighbours through any form of behaviour which could be considered offensive.

The anxieties of local people about the conduct of mentally handicapped neighbours vary from district to district and always reflect the attitudes current within their particular neighbourhood. Social customs in the south eastern counties of England, for example, differ markedly from those in the more northerly counties, and those in the West country from the communities in the Fen country.

Tolerance of lower standards of house and garden maintenance, of the style of dress of the residents, of drinking in the local pub and of sexual behaviour, will vary considerably and is dependent upon the past experience of any particular community and the composition of its residents. Only local knowledge can identify these attitudes.

Emotions tend to run high in any circumstances where people are placed in close propinquity with others not of their own choice. Keen suburban gardeners will resent a wild plant conservation plot next door to an immaculate garden, far more than other examples of non-conformist behaviour.

Loud radios or music playing at all hours will certainly offend older residents and parents with young children.

The fears of sexual misbehaviour are still evident when one discusses the possibility of mentally handicapped people living as neighbours, but these are more commonly expressed by older people than younger ones, a reflection of the more liberal attitudes currently held.

The identification of possible areas of sensitivity in any proposed scheme needs great care, and the training programme must include instruction in understanding the community attitudes appropriate to the area in which a group will live, as well as the basic life skills they will need for personal survival.

Any resident within a community needs to be on good terms with his neighbours if he is to be reasonably happy; the Chester Road scheme has evidently succeeded in this respect, for their people are well received by the practical, kindly inhabitants of a Midland working town. Accustomed to hard work, with memories of harsher times, sharing what is available with the less fortunate, the people of the West Midlands on the fringes of the Black Country have a sturdy independence which tolerates a scheme like the Chester Road project and does not see it as an immediate threat to their established way of life.

The philosophy of the Social Services staff most concerned with this venture is revealed in the views of two staff members. Ian Page, social work consultant in mental health to the County of Hereford and Worcester, states:

The training and preparation which takes place at Chester Road is geared very much towards helping mentally handicapped people to *handle their own affairs*, either as individuals, or in groups of two, three or four, depending on their needs and capacities. Groups are carefully chosen; some people are not as able as others to perform all the tasks necessary to enable them to live in the community happily and with dignity. Collectively, however, group members can combine their skills and cope well. Our general strategy, which we share with other agencies helping mentally handicapped people, is to enable them to live 'ordinary lives' in the community.

The senior social worker in Kidderminster, Roland Deakin, who is responsible for the Chester Road project, comments that, in his view, projects such as Chester Road are likely to fail unless there are sufficient numbers of professionally trained staff to provide the community supervision required for the objectives stated: mentally handicapped people 'managing their own affairs'.

For the Kidderminster residents, this implies paying rent and rates and other outgoings from their own budgets; shopping and cooking, just like others, to their own taste. This degree of independence can only be achieved by a very skilful and unobtrusive supervision, and Roland Deakin does not believe that this can be achieved by volunteers.

It is possible that in a busy working community, with a relatively small population of people of independent means – traditionally the providers of voluntary help in the past – those willing and able to give dependable and regular voluntary help, over long periods, are not so easily found. Earning a living is harder in the industrial areas; time is a valuable resource to be used in the main for personal essentials.

Whatever the reason, Roland Deakin sees the recruitment of additional trained staff as crucial to any further extension of the community living scheme on the Chester Road model.

He makes a second point regarding the content of the preparatory training: most people accepted into Chester Road have already received practical training in life skills, but have only theoretical knowledge of how these skills will be *applied* in independent living.

In many respects, social skills training is not as important as the development of inter-personal skills and learning to live with others. In our regular weekly meetings at Chester Road (attended by ex-Chester Road residents as well), we encourage residents to talk honestly about the emotional aspects of living together. Learning about sharing, decision-making, choosing, peace-making, confrontation and so on, is much more difficult.

The Chester Road team now cater for the six to eight people in training, plus twelve in houses and flats in the community, providing 24-hour cover. They envisage a constantly rising number of people requiring help and supervision as residents graduate from Chester Road.

The present staff establishment consists of one officer in charge and a deputy, both full time. Neither of these staff members is resident in Chester Road. They are assisted by two social workers, giving twenty hours each week, and a peripatetic social worker giving twenty-five hours a week, with support from the Social Services administrative department. This small staff undertakes all the individual training programmes in the preparation at Chester Road, negotiates housing in the community, assists residents to settle in and maintains close links with them thereafter, including the regular weekly meeting.

It may be helpful here to state that in social service parlance, the designation 'residential social worker' does not refer to the *function* of the staff member, but to his or her *qualification* as a person to work with those requiring residential help. None of those described as 'residential social worker' actually resides with the people they train or supervise. For this reason, the record book referred to earlier must be of great assistance in dealing with the everyday crises which arise as a result of less than usual ability or emotional stress. Staff members pass on to each other experience gained with members of the group and thus build up a very accurate picture of each individual's personality and ability.

The Chester Road project does not make use of volunteers in the planned programme towards independence. In the light of financial restrictions it may be that the further expansion of community living will depend upon an examination of all community resources to share the load. The initial programme and the individual training programmes certainly need professional guidance; but it is possible that some practical assistance could be provided for those resident in the community by other agencies, including voluntary organisations.

The skill and experience of those who initiate schemes is precious, and often incapable of duplication. The ability to decide which aspects of continuing care and supervision need professional skill, and which can be delegated to properly prepared helpers, may decide whether an imaginative scheme progresses and develops or is doomed to die in infancy, either when the originator leaves, or when there is a change in the policies of the authorities concerned.

The NIMROD Project – Cardiff

In 1975 a report on the development of future services for mentally handicapped people in the Cardiff area was submitted to the Welsh Office and the DHSS, and subsequently expanded in a working party report.

Plans for a comprehensive service for a population of approximately 60,000 people, were based on an estimated need of places for around 220 people who had been identified as requiring special provisions by virtue of mental handicap. Of these people, 55 were already in hospital or other institutional care, while the remainder were living at home. The ultimate objective, a home of their own within the community, was to be preceded by appropriate learning programmes for each individual. A central resource unit would provide facilities for meetings, leisure activities and a 24-hour emergency cover service.

The working party have stated their plans for community residences as follows:

Residential care. All NIMROD residential care will be provided in the community. Special efforts will be made to secure foster homes and lodgings and to ensure that the mentally handicapped people and their 'care families' receive full support. All the remaining residential accommodation will be provided in ordinary houses in the project catchment area. The houses are to be leased from Cardiff City Council who will purchase them and make them available at an economic rent. It is planned that six 'staffed houses' will eventually be established, each housing approximately six severely handicapped people. These will be fully staffed 24 hours a day. The work of care staff will be carefully planned to give the residents the opportunity to participate as fully as possible in normal daily activities and to be as independent as their handicap allows.

In addition, approximately four 'group houses' are planned. Four handicapped people will live in each house and receive the amount of support needed for independent community life. Although the group houses will not be staffed 24 hours a day, regular support will be provided by NIMROD domiciliary team members.

The planning and research, collection of evaluation data and the monitoring process began in June 1981, and was designed to select people to live in the first NIMROD Community.

Because the NIMROD project has a structured programme and defined objective, with a team of research officers and assistants under its Director, Roger Blunden, several detailed studies are scheduled for publication between 1982 and 1988.

The progress of this important pilot study will be of great interest to those engaged in planning community housing schemes for other areas, and the decision to release annual reports on all research aspects of NIMROD will enable a comparison to be made with other results without undue delay.

3 Housing Associations

The National Federation of Housing Associations is financed by the Government's Housing Corporation as a result of the Housing Act of 1974, which provided a charter for the Housing Association Movement. It sanctioned a series of grants for registered housing associations, to cover the net costs of approved new projects for the provision of dwellings for letting, or for hostels. The original objectives of the Housing Corporation were to provide ordinary homes to increase the housing stock provided by local authorities, for those in need and on modest incomes. It was not intended to provide for residences which required nursing or care staff to help or supervise the residents.

Only registered housing associations are entitled to public funds, and most are registered, via the Federation, with the Register of Friendly Societies. Currently, the number of homes provided by housing associations is well over a quarter of a million. Most of these provide subsidised rentals. They have an ongoing programme, financed by government grants and by loans through local authorities. Housing associations must have a management committee and are responsible to the Local Authority and the Housing Corporation for rent collection and maintenance of the properties, among other duties. Rents are fixed on a 'fair rent' basis by the Rent Officer, but all rebates on rent and rates available to ordinary council tenancies are also available to housing association tenants.

The criterion for tenancy is 'persons in necessitous circumstances upon terms appropriate to their means'. Some charitable housing trusts have specific requirements for tenancies – the elderly, or single working women, for example. In general, the housing associations have filled the gap left when private landlords left the field. They are particularly suited to·

the provision of homes for special local needs.

The Waltham Forest project, examined below, provides a detailed record over a period of years of a partnership with a housing association, which is still progressing and providing an increasing number of houses and flats.

The Waltham Forest Project

Waltham Forest is one of the outer London boroughs, with a population of 217,800. The area is bounded by Epping Forest and the River Lea, and contains large open expanses of forest land. The provision of homes in the community in this London Borough arose from the concern of a voluntary group, the Waltham Forest Local Society for Mentally Handicapped Children.

Parents in this area were concerned about the future of their mentally handicapped children, for whom the most probable residential facility was a mental handicap hospital in Essex, almost fifty miles outside the Borough.

The Local Society were fortunate in that their Chairman, Mr. Alex Sowerby, was employed in the architects' department of a local authority, and was thus familiar with statutory regulations. At that time many statutory services were being extended to provide improved services for mentally handicapped people, and the amendment to the Education Act of 1971 had begun to show itself in a wider use of educational resources for the benefit of children of members of the Society; but parents still saw, as their primary concern, the need to find alternatives to the hospital as a home for their children after their own deaths.

The parent members were familiar with the hospital conditions, and offered a service of voluntary help there. They estimated that there were a number of people in the wards who could live outside in the community if accommodation were provided, and some system of training and support designed. Accordingly, a local committee, the Outward Housing Group, was formed from members of the Society and other interested people, and they began to explore the possibility of providing houses through a partnership with a housing association.

There was already a local specialist housing association concerned with providing homes for elderly people; the Outward Group sought help and guidance from those concerned with this facility, and also consulted the Director of the National Federation of Housing Associations. It was decided not to form a new housing association to deal specifically with the needs of mentally handicapped people, but to join forces with an existing housing association, the Newlon Housing Trust.

When agreement had been reached on broad principles, it was arranged that properties would be acquired by Newlon and leased on a tenancy agreement to the Outward Group who would manage the properties, paying rent to Newlon. The Outward Group would be responsible for equipment and furniture and would carry out all the duties as agents of management of the properties.

Since the principal objective of the parents was to prevent the admission of their children to hospital, it was doubly fortunate that cordial relations with a consultant at the hospital already existed. Without the cooperation of the hospital staff, the idea of a pilot placement to test the hypothesis that mentally handicapped people could live outside the hospital would have proved impracticable.

It was obvious that, once the project had commenced, local support would be needed from the Social Services Department, and the Group accordingly approached the Director of Social Services and outlined their scheme. A member of the staff of the Social Services Department joined the Outward Group and acted as secretary. Later, representation of the Education Authority by a head teacher, and of the Area Health Authority by a psychologist, ensured professional advice on preparation and continuing support from these disciplines. The final composition of the steering committee was therefore a group of parents from the voluntary society (the initiators), members of the Newlon Housing Trust and the professionals mentioned above.

The importance was soon recognised of wholehearted cooperation by all those involved in the enterprise, and the multi-disciplinary composition of this committee contributed both strength and expertise to the initial stages and aided the harmonising of the inevitably opposing points of view. The resolution of such differences is an essential factor in the formation of a community project of this kind. The planning phase must involve compromise as the various elements – finance, staff, selection of properties, assessment of need, preparation of residents and the degree of supervision required – all come into question.

The Outward Group do not pretend that the period between the first purchase of properties, in late 1975, and the installing of the first independent group of people twenty-one months later, in 1977, was smooth sailing. The ideas were new, the training and preparation, theoretically well understood, had to be proven in practice.

No scientific test results can accurately measure the response of any individual, mentally handicapped or not, to a change of life style, nor predict the emotional response of one personality to another. The original plan was that all prospective residents should have a period of training in a house specially allocated for the purpose, with at least one resident staff member, and with instruction provided by the Adult Education Service. Six people were selected for training. Of mixed ages, they included two long-stay hospital residents, one from a hostel, and three who were currently living at home. The first property was converted to house this group, and over a period of nine months, as the reconstruction work proceeded, they received instruction in domestic and social skills.

This experience quickly demonstrated the importance of compatibility among those destined to live together. Unless the group are self-selected, and even if they are, temperament clashes, plain dislike and refusals to get on together must be expected and time allowed for adjustment. Some groups, however carefully assessed and selected, will simply not be able to live in harmony, and alternative accommodation will always be needed – if only for a short break – when people who have not lived together previously are required to do so.

When an established household loses one of its members, however, it may prove easier to introduce a new person, because a routine and balance between the group will already have been achieved; so the introduction of a replacement resident may not create the same degree of difficulty as was encountered when the initial group of four or so were shaking down together.

Such replacement may be easier if the new resident is known to the group, and is invited by them to join the household. This can happen when the existing group have all come from one hospital, or even one ward. On the other hand, difficulties may well arise if the existing group feel a replacement has been thrust upon them.

When planning a scheme of this kind, therefore, not only flexibility in the type and size of accommodation, but also provision for the inevitable vacancy replacements, are essential prerequisites for success. It is a good idea to maintain links between the units concerned, either by regular social meetings or by more formal sessions, so that interchange is always possible.

Contact should also be fostered between existing residents and possible future residents: those still in hospital, likely to be middle aged and over, and those at present living at home and attending schools or training centres. The example of people living successfully and independently in the community is a valuable training aid for those who will follow.

In 1977, while the first group were still finding their feet in a home of their own, the training house provided by the Local Health Authority became available and a structured course for independent living was devised.

A nurse was resident in the training house and the Adult Education Service provided instruction. A group of women were selected for instruction, and while they were living in the training house, the second group home was being purchased and converted. During the year the prospective residents were able to see the house and to choose wallpaper for their own rooms as well as deciding together on some of the decorations for the shared rooms. When they moved in, in March 1978, they had the support of a volunteer key person.

Mr. Alex Sowerby was closely involved with all this preliminary planning, and I quote from a paper he delivered in 1980, decribing the progress of the scheme at that time.

At this stage we took stock of our progress – painfully slow, with many problems, including the resignation of the Chairman of the Outward Committee on his departure from the district – but all concerned with Outward were as resolved as ever to continue.

It was always our intention to work towards providing a range of accommodation, from single person flats to supervised group homes.

We felt the quality of preparation training needed to be improved, and this was achieved by the willingness of the Social Services Department to approve two appointments to assist in the training and supervision at the training house.

Newlon Housing Trust were now in a position to provide the range of accommodation we required, so it was decided to proceed with the development of a scheme to assist the more dependent mentally handicapped person.

The Social Services Department agreed to establish a 'care person' post on a twenty hours per week basis, and a suitable property was acquired. A large back addition was to be converted into a maisonette for the 'care person', with access to the main part of the house which would be divided into two flats. It was decided that, as the future residents of the flats would be chosen from the Borough's hostels and would already have lived together for some time, they would receive their training from the care person when they moved in, instead of having a period of residence in the training house. This scheme would run concurrently with groups in training at the training house who would be moving on into their own homes.

Also at this stage, the role of the volunteer 'Key People', together with their back-up teams, was re-assessed. The quality of the volunteers and the commitment they were willing to make was excellent; the major concern was the amount of time each volunteer could give. The Social Services Department created the post of Group Homes Supervisor in September 1978, and appointed a woman experienced in Day Centre management, who was to play an important part in the future developments of the Outward Housing Group.

Prior to this appointment, a small terraced house was offered to Outward which would provide a very comfortable home for the next group in training – three women, all from different backgrounds and having an age range of 50 to 70 years. The house was ready for occupation in April 1979, and since moving in the occupants have been supported by resident helpers.

During the second half of 1979 a second training house came into operation, enabling two groups of five to begin training. In the first training house the group consisted of three men and two women, with an age range of 30–40 years. Three had been living in the local hostel, one in the local hospital and one at home. In the second training house, the group consisted of three women and two men – one woman aged 60 and the rest with an age range, like the first group, between 30 and 40 years. Their previous places of residence had been proportionally similar to those in the first training house.

Suitable houses were purchased for them, and meanwhile work on the home chosen for conversion into flats was completed. The care person and the residents moved in, two women being settled in one flat and two men and a woman in the other.

To complete the initial phase of the development, planning permission was granted for the conversion of a house into four bed-sitting rooms, each completely self-contained with a separate kitchen and bathroom. These units are now occupied.

Alex Sowerby comments:

There were many problems in the purchase and planning approval of this property, including the local Planning Department's concern regarding the off-street parking facilities and the possible number of car owners amongst the future residents, but this particular house was a 'natural' for this type of conversion. It was situated alongside a Methodist Church where several church members were keen to give a 'befriending' commitment to the future occupants.

We had decided to plan our development in phases, each phase itself providing as wide a range of different types of accommodation as possible. This would allow for some movement of residents, even though our basic philosophy was that we were offering a permanent home – 'their own home' – where one paid a visit by invitation, just like the people next door.

At the time of writing the first phase is now complete. It has taken six years to establish a housing stock comprising seven houses which contain twelve independent units providing accommodation for thirty-one mentally handicapped people, and two women are now living in single-person flats.

The provision of a second Group Homes Supervisor and one further care person has been agreed by the Local Authority to start in 1982. The importance of this commitment by the Social Services Department cannot be stressed too much, for without such cooperation, Outward Housing Group could not have developed in the way it has.

In Waltham Forest plans are being made for the individual housing needs of the future generation of mentally handicapped people wishing to live independently, with the current changes taken into account. Today, people entering the training homes are much younger, and there are significantly more men involved. Many of these people may wish to live on their own – in a bed-sitting room or flat – or, possibly, to share a flat with a friend. With these possibilities in mind, three further houses are being provided to be converted into small units – bed-sitting rooms, one and two-bedroom flats – with accommodation for a supporting staff member.

Alex Sowerby feels that so far the Outward Group have been involved in a catching up exercise, providing homes for people inappropriately housed in hospital. From the experience gained during the last seven years it is clear that a much wider range of provision will be required than just a basic group home where four or five mentally handicapped people live together. The role of the training houses is being re-examined with the Social Services Department.

It might be possible, for instance, to provide accommodation for foster parents who would be prepared to look after children.

At every stage of the Waltham Forest project the Outward

Group have been prepared to adapt and change in response to new factors. This flexibility is the key to their success.

The Social Services Department of Waltham Forest arranged for me to visit two of the houses provided by the Newlon Housing Trust.

I first met a group of four women living in a small terrace house in a quiet street, within walking distance of Leyton High Street. We talked in the comfortable sitting-room, and the social worker who introduced us was obviously a welcome and friendly visitor. This group of women were not all the original tenants; of the first four, all long term hospital patients, who had moved in after preparation, one of the younger women had graduated fairly quickly into a flat of her own. The three others had then invited a fourth woman, whom they had known for some time in hospital, to join them. Although advanced in years, she was still active, and the new group of four settled down well together.

The women have two main lines of contact for help: the Social Services Department, and a voluntary key worker from the Outward Housing Group which manages the house. The social workers are not normally available after office hours or at weekends, except in emergencies, but the voluntary key worker accepts an all-round cover.

Both this visit and the subsequent one revealed aspects of community living which are worth consideration and which will require thought in setting up similar housing units. For instance, I learned that the older woman, who had joined the group from the hospital, had died suddenly after eighteen months of residence. One of the other women found her dead in the bathroom and, by mischance, the social worker was out of the office on another visit when they telephoned.

However, the three women dealt with the situation in a practical manner, contacting neighbours and the local police, and showing themselves well able to come to terms with the fact of death and its concomitant arrangements. The situation was eased by the fact that the woman who died had a niece. She was able to handle the funeral arrangements, and all the remaining women attended the service. The simple rituals of death and bereavement are part of life experience, and mentally handicapped people living like others will inevitably share these experiences with us.

The three friends were then joined by a fourth woman in her late fifties. She was a local resident who had lived with an elderly mother. Fortunately, as the mother became more frail, she had arranged for her daughter to spend time, one day a week, in the training house, and when she was finally admitted to the hospital where she died, another daughter was able to care for her mentally handicapped sister and to see her through the immediate period of grieving.

Now, six months later, this mentally handicapped woman lives comfortably with the group. Her sister is quite near and visits regularly, and is visited in turn.

This close family and neighbourhood contact obviously contributes to the security and normality of the residents. Because their hospital had been in a nearby area, existing family ties had been maintained and helped to ease the process of adjustment to community life.

The sense of belonging to a place and to a family is obviously a deeply felt human need. While people live in the hospital, the institution itself is 'home' – familiar, if not ideal – and each resident has a place and achieves some identity with the group as a whole. When they leave this secure environment, there must of necessity be a period of confusion and a need to re-identify with new conditions.

Each fresh experience forces the group to re-align itself to cope with the new conditions. The experience of death, and the exposure to the role of the family in such situations, had caused one of the older women in the group to attempt to contact her own family. She told me that she had been sent into hospital as a very young child and had no family contact since.

The social worker was trying to trace her family from a search of the register of births, and this was obviously a source of interest and some anxiety to her. The other three residents all had family links; one indeed, was away on a weekend visit at the time I was with them.

Conversations reveal many long-felt wants. It emerged during the discussion that this lady had never known when her birthday was and, during her years as a child, had never had a birthday party. Her memory may not have been reliable, but the woman who had most recently joined the group, on the death of her own mother, was clearly distressed at the thought of these lost childhood pleasures which she had herself enjoyed; she told me that she thought it was 'a terrible thing – not to have a birthday card or a present.' The woman who was seeking her family recounted her memories of the years in hospital in a matter of fact way, as a remembrance of old times, without undue bitterness. She said, 'If they find my brothers and sisters, they might not want to know. Could be bad, could be good.'

It is obvious that the links with families are very important to residents coming late into community life, and they should not be ignored in the programme of preparation. Social skills include dealing with the emotions of family living, good and bad, and if these have been severed early in life, and are to be forged in later years, some adjustment will be inevitable. Not everyone will wish to be reminded, after a lapse of years, that they have a handicapped brother or sister whom, in many cases, they have never seen. In this instance, the young social worker, while doing all she could to discover if this woman had any living relatives, was also carefully preparing her for possible disappointments.

The third woman in the group was concerned about a notice of state benefit which had reached her and was reassured by the social worker that it was a formality and that no action was needed.

In the houses managed by the Outward Group the weekly payments cover rent, rates and heating. These are collected by the volunteer management group, and a controlled rent is paid over to the Newlon Housing Trust. There is an allowance in the rent for internal decoration. Anxieties over saving for heating and other outgoings are removed from this group, in comparison with the Kidderminster residents who are required to budget separately for these items.

Any financial worry in either group is really unnecessary; four incomes are more than adequate to deal with the expenses of ordinary homes. Each of the Waltham Forest housing units have coin box telephones (many ex-hospital residents derive great pleasure from the use of the telephone) and the need to put coins into the box does provide some check on the use of the telephone and the resulting heavy accounts.

As I have mentioned, once residents have graduated from the training house they no longer have 24-hour access to social services staff. During their period of residence in the training house, they are able to call the non-resident responsible staff in their own homes at any time, but out in the community, this cover is provided by the volunteer 'key person'.

My second call was made to a young man, newly installed in a house which had been converted into four self-contained flats. He had spent the previous six years since the death of his father, his last surviving parent, in other Outward accommodation.

He made us some tea, and as we sat in his comfortable room I noticed that he was limping and in some apparent discomfort. It transpired that he had suffered an injury to both feet some years before, which resulted in the amputation of the toes of both feet.

He had attended his general practitioner's surgery three weeks previously and had been referred to hospital, where the amputation area on the affected foot was dressed, and he was due to attend again 48 hours after our visit. The social worker or a volunteer would accompany him on this visit, and would presumably be able to liaise with the general practitioner to ensure that any necessary home nursing treatment was carried out.

This young man had been provided with a modest inheritance by his father, enabling him to furnish his flat comfortably. Later, the social worker explained to me that his small capital sum was nevertheless more than that permitted as a level for supplementary benefit and that they had had to take steps to inform the authorities concerned.

This highlights another area of concern for those who must advise people coming from hospitals. The issue of 'patients' money' – savings accrued from allowances, discussed earlier by Dr. Geoffrey Harris – reminds parents who wish to provide for their mentally handicapped family members that even a modest level of inheritance may provide additional problems when supplementary benefits are needed.

This house, providing four units, will enable some hospital residents to live alone for the first time in their lives. One woman, living in the flat above the one I visited, was celebrating her independence by spending most of the morning in bed – a luxury denied her during many years of institutional living.

It is the opportunity to make possible such small acts of independence that inspires projects like the Outward Housing Group. Fighting to surmount all obstacles and objections, they have the reward of restoring, in small measure, some of the lost years to people who, through no fault of their own, have been denied an ordinary freedom.

4 Hostels and Group Homes

Since the mid-sixties there have been a number of pilot projects for various types of community residence. The voluntary organisations, particularly parent-oriented groups, were pioneers in this area. My long association with Mencap has obviously made me well aware of the work of the Local Societies, many of which provided houses of different kinds, from short-stay hostels designed to give parents a break, to permanent homes set up in partnership with housing associations and local authorities.

The concept of a real home – an ordinary house in an ordinary street, tenanted by a mentally handicapped person on the same terms as his neighbours – has arisen from the proposal to move people from mental handicap hospitals advocated in the White Paper of 1971, *Better Services for the Mentally Handicapped.* Those Local Authorities which accepted the responsibility for local hospital residents returned to their care began by building hostels to receive them. Some had as many as forty places, and often took people of one sex only, men in one house, women in another, with resident staff. Under such conditions, one institution was merely exchanged for another, albeit improved.

In the private sector, some commercial guest houses and small hotels leaped in to fill the immediate gap in available accommodation. Mentally handicapped people, decanted into the community after years of residence in hospital, without preparation and without any planned destination, were ripe for exploitation of all kinds.

Some establishments, while running on a profit making basis, genuinely attempted to give their residents an improved quality of life, but without professional knowledge or adequate support they could not offer any real semblance of independent community life. Many encountered hostile reactions from neighbours, who resented the sight of mentally handicapped people wandering aimlessly about the streets all day, totally unequipped to lead a useful life.

This pattern, repeated throughout the country, forced local authorities to consider making residential provision by building new hostels or converting existing premises. Since the people for whom these provisions were made had been discharged from institutions once expected to be permanent, it was perhaps natural that the idea of the hostel was also seen as a permanent solution in some cases. For many mentally handicapped people, without family ties and without experience of independent living, the hostel appeared likely to be a final home, with the prospect of a return to the hospital when age or infirmity gave rise to problems of care which the hostel could not provide.

At the time of the Mental Health Act of 1959, public health authorities were part of the local government service and were responsible for the provision of centres and facilities for the training and occupation of mentally handicapped people. Accommodation and residential care was, in the main, provided by the local mental hospital. The local authority concerned itself chiefly with Junior Training Centres for 'ineducable' children – those with IQs under 50 – and with Adult Training Centres for those over school age, at that time, 15 years.

Hostels were included in the ten-year plan for England and Wales, published in 1962, but by the time of the publication of the 1971 White Paper, only 4,850 hostel places had been provided, and many of these were much larger than the 30-place unit (15 male and 15 female) which Mencap had planned as a model in Slough.

The re-organisation of the National Health Service in 1970 transferred the responsibility for local authority services for mentally handicapped people to the Social Services Departments, excluding education, and there has been a gradual increase in the past ten years in provisions for residence in the community. By 1974, the consultative document *Priorities in the Health and Social Services in England* gave the number of places for mentally handicapped people, provided by local authorities, private and voluntary homes, as over 9,500. There were still more than

55,000 in hospital, and mentally handicapped babies were still being born. The numbers of children quoted in 1972 as being in special educational need because of mental handicap were around 80,000 mildly mentally handicapped and 33,000 severely mentally handicapped (*Mental Handicap – Ways Forward*, O.H.E., 1978).

Clearly, forward planning for the ultimate housing of the large group of people currently living in the community was a matter of urgent concern. (A small number of severely handicapped children were still resident in hospitals and attending hospital schools run by the Education Authority; their numbers appear within the 33,000.)

The Cherries Project

Group homes gradually emerged as the next step, and local authorities often made forward plans for both hostels and group homes of different sizes; in the early stages these were planned as single sex homes, and few were designed for an average sized family group. In many cases resident staff accommodation was provided to give 24-hour surveillance.

One of the earlier projects was the Cherries Group Home in Berkshire, the subject of a study by D. G. and D. M. Race, published by HMSO in 1979. They give a detailed account of the changes in public awareness which resulted in the idea of 'trainable' mentally handicapped people, and their ability to be employed in some limited capacity in simple industrial work. The general acceptance of full employment for all, and the consequent merit of productive labour, was used as a measure of the value of an individual, to be set against the cost to society of caring for those unable to contribute.

The Cherries project, begun by the Buckingham Social Services Department, requested nominations from the Slough Mencap Society for ten places to be allocated in the new group home. From the beginning, the project was intended to be fully researched as a feasibility study, to see if mentally handicapped adults of varying mental ability could live without supervision, and the DHSS assisted with the funding on this premise.

The final report of the period from 1973 to 1976 is detailed and will repay full study. The conclusion of the researchers is that the hostel is currently serving as a 'half-way house' between staffed accommodation and council housing. They add that they are not totally convinced of the need for such a half-way house situation and believe that, at least for adults like those resident at the Cherries, who were working in the community at that time, small self-contained flats, converted from the hostel building, would solve the problems inevitable in a house for twelve persons, either staffed or unsupervised. Their conclusions have been borne out by experiences elsewhere.

Some authorities do provide a 'training home' both for people from hospital accommodation and for those leaving private households on the death of parents, but increasingly it is seen to be as simple to give any necessary additional instruction actually in the living accommodation provided, whether flat or council house, since many of the residents have already received 'life skills' instruction.

The inevitable tendency to lapse into jargon has led me to ponder on the terms 'life skills' and 'social skills'. Both embrace the skills of living with others and personal survival. I noticed, however, in the places I visited for this book that 'life skills' are generally interpreted as survival techniques, cooking for and feeding oneself and others, hygiene, use of money and other practical needs, whereas 'social skills' are concerned with emotional responses. There is a tendency to regard the practical skills as the province of the helpers from the hospital, nursing and community health services, and the emotional skills as the perquisite of social work. I regard this division as unlikely to produce the best results for mentally handicapped people.

Planning and cooking a meal for a group can produce emotional crises just as often as adolescent sexual experiments. On a visit to a Canadian Adult Centre which was concerned in training mentally handicapped people for open employment, I was told that the instructor/chef introduced a session of 'creative temperament' into his teaching sessions. 'All chefs go mad at times,' was his philosophy, 'throw pans and scream; the kitchen staff have to get used to it.' There are no experts in human emotions, and the behaviourists are often observers only.

Mentally handicapped people preparing to live together as a group have the same difficulties in initial adjustments as others, and from their past experience gradually achieve a balance which assists them to return to the norm of behaviour after a crisis. Too much well-meant analysis may actually be harmful to the process of emotional development.

The least able mentally handicapped person will always require help and supervision. In practice, others in the group can usually provide what is needed and know when to ask for help in a situation which is beyond their power to solve.

The hostel situation will usually require staff resident, simply because the sum of a number of problems placed in propinquity will always be greater than the sum of the parts involved. Twelve severely handicapped people living together will present difficulties in management additional to the twelve individuals concerned. On the other hand, the small unit, made up of complementary people, may well reduce the initial problems presented by a difficult member, because the group will modify the anti-social behaviour by their own methods.

Describing 'group homes', C. E. Gathercole states categorically that, whether staffed or not, the number of residents should not exceed five or six mentally handicapped people. Of the places I have seen, homes with more than four residents were usually training units, with the occupation of a flat or council house as the ultimate objective. Chris Gathercole also states that he sees the need for staff only for those who are profoundly handicapped or have additional physical handicaps. He makes the point that 'ordinary homes are more likely to offer opportunities for learning skills for independent living than segregated institutions'. They certainly offer better opportunities for *practice* of learned skills, which alone can produce proficiency.

The Expansion of Group Home Projects

During the past ten years there have been several studies of accommodation needs. Two of these are the results of voluntary effort on a local basis. High Wycombe Society for Mentally Handicapped Children published their findings in 1980 and concentrated upon the future needs of the 182 people currently living at home with their own families. 120 were still in school, the 98 people in Adult Training Centres lived mainly at home and only 31 were living in hostel accommodation. It is interesting that in their conclusions they envisage that an average of nine additional people annually over the next five years will need to be taken into care by the Social Services because their families will no longer be able to look after them at home; they propose an additional *hostel* of 30 places as a solution, and the provision of group or satellite homes as a *secondary* solution for permanent care.

The second study in the South East Region of the Royal Society for Mentally Handicapped Children – *Home Sweet Home?* – looked at village communities, hostels, hospital units, co-resident homes, sheltered housing and commercial boarding houses. They conclude that 'while welcoming the increased provision of small, local units, in ordinary houses', they 'emphasise the importance of isolation of such units', and continue: 'Unless they are integrated into a system of residential provision, *staff* will lack the support and stimulus of outside contacts, the stability of the home may be threatened and residents denied opportunities for alternative placements, should the present one be inappropriate.' The study group are much concerned about this problem and suggest that voluntary organisations which provide accommodation 'need to get together to explore ways in which the voluntary homes can be linked to the statutory scheme of residential provision.'

When a local group decides that there is a need for a small group home, and commences with a partnership with a local authority, as both the Wyre Forest and Waltham Forest groups have done, in different ways, the link is there from the start.

This study conceives the group home as a permanent 'home', with staff supervision from a 'parent' hostel, providing regular weekly contact, or supervision from an identified field social worker. They see the need for 24-hour cover as essential for the independent home, but emphasise that privacy for the residents should preclude an overload of visitors.

The report contains a list of the factors which the group decided were to be evaluated in deciding whether the amenity studied was good or lacking in some essentials, and they list the homes visited, which were situated in widely different areas.

There are at least two group homes which are shared by both mentally handicapped people and non-handicapped people: the Cardiff University Social Service Group Home, which has five mentally handicapped people living with three non-handicapped adults; and L'Arche, Lambeth, which has eight mentally handicapped adults with three or four non-handicapped adults. Chris Heginbotham, in his *Housing for Mentally Handicapped People* (1980), describes two homes: one shared by five mentally handicapped adults and two able bodied adults who work locally and support the group, and the second by three mentally handicapped people and two able bodied tenants. The experiences of the Camden Society with group homes suggests that the 'able tenant model' is more suited to the more able mentally handicapped group, and the severely handicapped residents would need greater assistance from professionally trained staff.

Chris Heginbotham, as Area Manager of a Housing Association, Circle 33 Housing Trust Ltd., reports on the difficulties as well as the successes of group homes, and in his 1981 report, *Housing Projects for Mentally Handicapped People*, comments in detail, with actual plans and elevations, on six projects of widely different types, sharing valuable experience with those who wish to plan for the future.

He says 'we must guard against assuming that mentally handicapped people need something "special" just because they are mentally handicapped rather than, say, because they are on low incomes or have a learning difficulty.' His report has features which can apply equally to other groups, such as housing for elderly people, students or other homeless individuals. Special needs for housing cover many people and there are funds for this purpose. Chris Heginbotham reminds us that because some groups have a 'special need' it may not mean that the supplying of that need requires a 'special' house or flat.

Many group homes have been initiated by the local societies of Mencap, and later handed over to the Social Services Departments of the areas concerned. As one example, the Mencap Coventry Society purchased an end of terrace house in 1978, with funds which had taken over ten years to raise, and provided a home of their own for four men who had lived in a hostel nearby. The residents are self-supporting, sharing the costs of running the home and looking after themselves well. Much of the success of their venture into independence is attributed to the preparation they received in the hostel. Their transfer into a community-based home has released places for others to be similarly prepared.

In Avon, too, the principle of using the hostel as a half-way house to independent living is established. The group home itself may be a stage towards living in a flat alone or with one other tenant. Writing on these policies in 1979, Steve Howell, a specialist social worker concerned with group homes says, 'There will be vacancies in group homes from time to time – for example when tenants marry and move into council flats. There is no reason why these vacancies cannot be filled directly from the community' (for example, from adults living at home). 'We need to develop an elastic system, responsible to need as an alternative to residential care. The beauty of such a scheme is that you need little or no purpose-built accommodation and with proper training the social work and community nursing supervision need not be obtrusive.'

In 1976, Vince Gorman, Divisional Nursing Officer, North-gate Hospital, Morpeth, reporting on the 60,000 adults and children at that time in hospital care, said that in his view a hostel of twenty to thirty places was a mini-institution. Alternative residences should be in the smallest group setting possible, and should be sited in the local communities of mentally handicapped people.

The Need for Housing
Those most closely concerned with mentally handicapped people, parents and professionals from all disciplines, have long seen the objective of independent living within the community as the only real future alternative to the continuation of the large mental handicap hospital, and have planned and organised training schemes to this end. All this effort will be frustrated unless we begin at the *other* end and commence *now* to make

available a fair share of housing to be occupied by mentally handicapped people after proper preparation.

Hostels are now choc-a-bloc with residents for whom no alternatives are available, and adult mentally handicapped people living at home must continue to do so for want of an interim hostel place. Increasingly, Adult Training Centres, or Social Education Centres as they may now be designated, have to refuse further admissions because there is no 'graduation' from a training centre or the hostel accommodation designed for students or 'trainees' at the Centre.

This situation has arisen because of the failure to face squarely the *ultimate* residential need of mentally handicapped people. Although they comprise the largest *single* group of disabled people, their numbers in any local authority district will be assessable and manageable, with good forward planning, which should be based upon the numbers now in special education because of mental handicap, and not based upon waiting lists for adult centres or hostels.

If parents with mentally handicapped children approaching adult life were to place their names on local authority housing lists as requiring homes, at least the authority could plan on placing them in groups of four or five and, numerically at least, estimate the ultimate allocation of ordinary homes required. Their preparation could then also be planned progressively and the need for additional expensive purpose-built amenities reduced. The group home of mixed ability tenants, of both sexes in most cases, will probably prove the best solution for the future, if the experience of the past ten years is any guide.

Supervision can take many forms, but increasingly it becomes obvious that whilst professional back-up is needed for particular difficulties, what is needed by mentally handicapped people who have achieved an independent life in the community today is nothing more nor less than an intelligent friend, who is also a near neighbour.

People who have been housed in homes of their own after having lived with their parents need a different approach from hospital groups, because people who have lived in the community may not need the intensive preparation which is necessary for those who have lived in institutions. They are familiar with their environment, they are familiar with the public services of the neighbourhood, transport and shops, and are able to function adequately. Many of them can read enough to recognise familiar signs; some of them read sufficiently well to be able to enjoy a newspaper or a magazine; others read well enough to enjoy borrowing books from the library. In other words, they are already prepared to live in the community. The tragedy in the past has been that on the death of their parents, there were few alternatives to the admission to the large institution where many of the skills which had been patiently acquired over the years were lost.

The Homes Foundation Scheme

Recognising that even the best preparatory training for community life is useless unless there is a real prospect of a home in the future, the parent members of the Royal Society for Mentally Handicapped Children and Adults commissioned a feasibility study on the possibility of their family members continuing to live in their own homes after the parents' death.

Many parents owned their own homes, but lacked enough other financial resources to ensure a future for their mentally handicapped children, comparable to that which they had enjoyed at home.

The prospect for their mentally handicapped sons or daughters, of eventual admission to a mental handicap hospital for the rest of their lives, was a constant source of distress to parents who had battled for years to enable them to live at home.

The study of needs and resources resulted in the setting up of a Homes Foundation by MENCAP, in April 1982. The scheme is in its infancy, and the aims and objectives, the legal, financial and management structure, are set out in a detailed document. The plan will be modified by experience, and each family will need to consider their own situation and be guided by the advice of their own solicitor. The Homes Foundation has been designed as a service to parents, supported by the national organisation; the help of professional staff is available when setting up a local project, but it is made clear that the initiative and impetus must come from the people on the spot.

It is vital to stress that Homes Foundation projects will only be able to operate in those areas where the Local Society is prepared to take an active and enthusiastic part in planning, creating and maintaining the home. This is not a scheme that will be – or should be – run entirely by the Royal Society from its London Headquarters. Local supervision and support, and active cooperation with Social Services and Health, are the keys to the successful development of projects. Parents who are interested should therefore first contact their own Local Society to see what plans are being made.

The emergence of self-help schemes such as this is due to the realisation of urgent need which is unlikely to be filled in time by statutory sources. Parents have seen the great improvements made by appropriate education of their children, resulting in a maximisation of their abilities. They are concerned to obtain continued education in adult life to maintain this improvement, and they are concerned to ensure that their children will not be forced into hospital care for lack of community provisions.

5 Conclusions

It must be obvious that the success of any project will depend upon the cooperation of the Local Authority. The physical provision of the houses will come from the housing stock provided by council housing, or by housing associations which are linked to the council provision. The supervisory services will come from the Social Services Department and without the wholehearted support of the Local Authority concerned no scheme will get off the ground.

In many local authorities today there are schemes similar to those examined above. They have many elements in common, and with the wide range of abilities among the mentally handicapped people they serve, all will have common problems: the need for training, for professionally qualified people to identify training needs and devise individual programmes, flexible housing units designed to serve people with varying needs and, above all, the need to plan ahead at every stage, so that no project is brought to a halt by a bottle-neck situation which has not anticipated inevitable changes.

But each area will likewise have elements unique to its own neighbourhood, and these will dictate, first of all, the community reaction to the way in which mentally handicapped people are to be received and where they will live.

For this reason, it is well-nigh impossible to select any one project as, to use the fashionable jargon, 'an example of excellence', or a 'model of good practice'. The scheme which is best suited to the needs and resources of a particular area will achieve the best standard of reasonable happiness for the mentally handicapped residents, and give the best value for the money spent to provide it.

Life within the community is not trouble-free for any of us. If mentally handicapped people are to share this life with us, they will experience the trials and tribulations common to us all. What does emerge from the visits I have made is that they are as capable as the rest of us at dealing with the ordinary hazards that arise. The group in the West Midlands coped with appalling winter conditions, the worst for years, digging out their front paths, getting to their daily work, handling very difficult and disturbed members of the family group, and achieving a real stability which supported them in crises.

The elderly ladies in Waltham Forest, confronted with sudden death, were saddened and shocked, but not overthrown by the experience.

We have much to learn of the capacity for survival of mentally handicapped people. It has sometimes seemed to me that the marked deficiency in highly intelligent people of that quality we call 'common sense', is compensated by an additional measure of it in mentally handicapped people.

A little self-examination will often reveal the extent to which we tend to underestimate mentally handicapped people. For example, during one of my visits, one lady asked where I lived. I replied that on occasion I had to have accommodation in London in order to work during the week in the office, although my home was elsewhere. She replied, not unnaturally, that having two places to keep must be very expensive. My initial reaction was surprise that she should have so instantly assessed the crucial point; my second was to reprove myself for being surprised. My friends and acquaintances would not have made the comment, for a variety of reasons. She made it not only because it was obvious, but because she wished to express her understanding and sympathy. The spontaneous understanding by mentally handicapped people of many situations is not fully credited to them because they do not always express what they feel. We are so used to concealing emotions, deducing from past experience what is acceptable and what is not, that we fail to recognise the contribution which mentally handicapped people could make to the solution of some of their own problems by more simple and direct responses to them, and particularly to each other.

What does emerge, as a common factor, is the absolute need for the total cooperation of all concerned and the full understanding of community resources; particularly the role of housing associations in partnership with local authorities.

The earlier sections of this book were concerned with the preparation of mentally handicapped people for independent living within the community and dealt with two main groups: long-stay hospital residents, and young people of school-leaving age who have been cared for by their families. But in every community there will be groups of mentally handicapped people of all ages, from different backgrounds and with different abilities, and they will also need preparation.

No matter how excellent the training provided, all such work is useless unless at the end of it there is real hope that homes will be made available. The official view, that 15,000 people currently in mental handicap hospitals could be enabled to live in the community if homes were provided, assumes that around 4,000 houses are needed throughout the country for this group alone.

If hospital admissions were to cease completely – an unrealistic supposition – there would still remain the problem of future housing provision for those currently living at home; it cannot be presumed that they will live with their families in their present home for the rest of their lives.

The review *Mental Handicap: Progress, Problems and Priorities* by Peter Mittler, published by the DHSS in 1980, suggests that at present 70% of severely mentally handicapped children between the ages of 5–15 live at home. By the time they reach the age group 16–44, only 40% are still living with their families, and by the age of 45 and over the percentage has fallen to only 10%.

These estimates – for the report stresses that the figures are approximate only – would appear to confirm the view that whilst families cope reasonably well with children during the school years, when faced with young adults in the family home all day, without occupation or continuing education, parents are under increased pressure to find alternative accommodation. If this is not available in the locality, admission to a mental handicap hospital may be the only solution.

The problem of accommodation for older mentally handicapped people becomes acute as their parents age or die. If they have not received education in independent living and they are unable to look after themselves, the training required in self-care, cooking, independent travel and other essential skills for life in the community, may well defeat those who accept their care. Equally, those who have functioned well in their own neighbourhood, know the locality and are known by other residents, may have great difficulty and experience real distress when confronted by a move to a distant hostel or mental handicap hospital and speedily regress to dependence.

The community is not only faced with providing for those at present in hospital who could be moved out, but with continuing provision for those who are now infants, school children, young adults and ageing mentally handicapped people – all of whom are being cared for by their families and are thus accustomed to a family life style.

Today the emphasis in Training Centres is shifting from the older work-orientated form of occupational training, into education in the skills of self-care and social usage.

Many local authorities have provided increasing assistance from the education service to the instructors and staff of Training Centres; indeed, some are now designated 'Social Education Centres'. But to teach mentally handicapped young adults to cook and garden, to tackle laundry and house maintenance and to manage a simple household budget, is to raise their hopes and expectations of living in a home of their own, like other people. Without ensuring that this is possible of attainment, it is as cruel as training them for outside employment by the use of simple contract work, during a period of recession and high unemployment.

Training for living, for mentally handicapped people no less than the rest of us, means training for life as it really is, according to future provisions and possibilities. At present, it would appear more realistic to offer those approaching their mid-forties courses in how to survive in a mental handicap hospital, for the chances are that they will end their days there after the death of their parents. The contribution of local authority education and social services departments will be wasted endeavour, unless a similar commitment can be made by the housing departments.

Education for everyone today is facing rapid change. The influence of the micro-chip must result in increased leisure, and simple home management has become an essential do-it-yourself activity. Mentally handicapped residents will need to know how to carry out redecorating, undertake simple repairs, maintain their gardens and deal with refuse disposal, just like the rest of the community.

They will need education for leisure; to learn how to make use of local facilities for sports and other hobbies and how to use the services provided by public libraries; and they will need to understand and accept the responsibilities of community life, as well as enjoying the rights of citizens, if they are to become truly independent citizens.

So planning must work *backwards*, from the allocation of adequate housing to the programmes and physical resources needed to prepare mentally handicapped people to occupy these units, be they single-person flats or shared homes for five or six people who choose to live together as a family group.

The process must be continuous, for a home is a home for life where most mentally handicapped people are concerned. Every year more people will require accommodation, at least until preventive research materially affects the incidence of mental handicap within the population. As matters stand today, advances in medical care and pharmacology have ensured the survival even of those with severe degrees of handicap, and have thus increased the prevalence within the community. Mental handicap is not a condition which will vanish in the foreseeable future.

Proper planning and enlightened provision can minimise the problems which have arisen from inappropriate treatment in the past. Flexibility is essential; each local authority has factors which are unique to itself, and no centrally designed scheme can take all the variables into account. Statutory funding, and local funds, can be applied in many different ways and in many combinations, to provide what is needed in a particular area.

The individual good will and enterprise which has marked so many of the projects studied should not be stifled by any purely bureaucratic controls. The approach should be to define the need, design how it should be met and then apply common sense to provide it, in the way which will give best value to the community as a whole, as well as to the mentally handicapped individual.

The consultative document *Care in the Community*, published by the DHSS in July 1981, suggests that an allocation of £68.5 million for the period 1981-82, and of £71 million for 1982-83, be made to Joint Finance funding for patient care – that is for projects jointly administered by the NHS and local authorities. Of this it is estimated that about 33% is for mental handicap projects.

Both local authorities and voluntary bodies sponsored by local authorities can receive funding for initial capital costs and for revenue costs in the first three years, with an extension for a further four years. There is, however, a proviso that when such projects are planned it must be accepted that, at the conclusion of the period of financial aid, the cost of continuing the project will be borne by the local authority.

These joint fund ventures are intended to relieve the hospitals of health care, including residence for patients, and do not provide for local authority housing. However, they *may* do so for people who are transferred from hospital to social service care.

It should not be beyond the bounds of possibility to design schemes for hospital discharges which could include some ordinary houses, perhaps including a percentage of homes with a few modifications – extra-wide doors and larger kitchens and bathrooms, with adapted fixtures – which would make it possible for handicapped people to live comfortably in ordinary council houses.

Most authorities provide housing for elderly people as an essential part of their planning; the disabled should equally be considered. Mentally handicapped people *are* disabled, but in the main they do not need specially designed homes; residences allocated from the regular housing stock are usually adequate for their needs.

Today most mentally handicapped people are in receipt of statutory benefits which cover their reasonable expenses. If three or four live together, their joint incomes are more than sufficient to pay for the rent, rates and running costs of an ordinary house. Moreover, as I saw so clearly when I visited them in their own homes, they are more than capable of managing their own finances and living comfortably with their neighbours.

PART FOUR

Planning for the Future

1 The Need for Organised Planning

For mentally handicapped people the progress towards independent life in the community is dependent upon many factors, some of them fixed and irrevocable, but many more subject to the ebb and flow of the tides of public opinion and economic instability. Like the tides, the advances and retreats are occasionally subject to tremendous surges, which gain territories in new and unexplored areas. When the impetus of this surge fades, the gains may be lost, or they may be consolidated by seizing the opportunities thus provided for extension beyond previous boundaries.

The promulgation by the WHO of the Rights of Mentally Handicapped People was such a surge, brought about by the patient continual pressure over many years by the families of those concerned. It resulted in a widening of public acceptance of the duty to provide services and, in the optimism of the time, the anticipation of the financial ability to do so.

As the economic situation worsened, postponement of objectives became the rule rather than the exception in all services, but the tide was slowly mounting towards the next great surge, and manifested itself in an outbreak of public investigation – and public outcry – into the conditions prevailing in mental handicap hospitals. The result was the realisation that mental handicap was a problem which could no longer be tidied away.

The ground gained is now under consolidation; life in the community for the disabled is seen to be their right, and modifications by the community to enable disabled people to live with others is recognised as a duty. It is now increasingly common, for example, for shops, places of entertainment, toilets and other facilities, to provide wheelchair access. Electrically propelled chairs and small cars which enable completely immobilised people to use the pavements of cities to shop are no longer a rare sight. Many programmes on the media, both sound and visual broadcasting, as well as reports in the Press, are daily advancing the cause of mentally handicapped people who today live among us in their families, in hospitals and in hostels.

What should we be contemplating for the future, and how can it be achieved?

The results of a most important surge towards new territories, the Education Act, Handicapped Pupils, 1970, are not yet fully realised.

For more than ten years the education services of local authorities have provided for even the most severely mentally handicapped child to receive appropriate education. Most are now able, at school leaving age, to care for their own physical needs and are acquiring, in early adolescence, the additional skills needed for living in the community. Parents have had their role acknowledged as partners in the teaching process and increasingly participate in individual programmes to improve areas in which their child needs special help, often identified by the parents themselves.

What kind of home?

Those concerned with the provision for adult life of the young person who has been prepared for independent living are all agreed on the need for flexibility of residential amenities.

The Family Home

There will be some mentally handicapped people who wish to continue to live with their parents for as long as those parents remain alive; and there will be some parents, particularly single parents through desertion, divorce or the death of their partners, who may wish to have the mentally handicapped member to live with them on the same terms; there are some brothers and sisters of mentally handicapped people who receive them into their own homes after their marriages and do not see this as a burden.

It is important to avoid a rigid value judgement in all these situations. Over-protection is frequently alleged against parents who still keep mentally handicapped adults at home with them, but in some cases this may result in the greatest possible degree of happiness for the affected person, even if at the end it means grief when the parent dies and there is the upsetting experience of a move from the family home. We cannot make a logical, balanced assessment, setting years of content against eventual trauma, nor are we qualified to use the yard-stick of our own desire for early and complete independence to measure what might be appropriate for others.

Most of the planned projects are based upon the imitation of a close family group, so it would seem that this is the model which is favoured. It is not sensible, therefore, to destroy a functioning family group which is satisfactory to both generations and seek to remove *all* mentally handicapped people to hostels or group homes as they become adult.

Hostel Accommodation

Nor is it sensible to decry *all* lodging arrangements on the grounds of possible exploitation of mentally handicapped lodgers. Even some non-handicapped lodgers are certainly exploited, but others are perfectly content to spend some part of their lives, often in their early working years, with a kindly landlady. In general, mentally handicapped people are less likely to be exploited because they will usually have social services supervision. Hostel life will suit some people very well; they may not wish to be concerned with individual participation in all aspects of housekeeping and daily social intercourse with different neighbours, preferring a structured environment and known companions; after all, people of both sexes voluntarily enter the religious life which is the epitome of a sharing community.

If mentally handicapped people are to be granted the same range of choice, acknowledging differences of ability, of temperament, emotions and the changing needs of life, many types of accommodation will be needed, but all must have a clearly designed purpose.

In the past some of the worst problems have arisen because of failure to define the purpose of a particular provision. Hospitals are normally expected to cure, or at least alleviate, a medical condition. Hospitals for chronically sick people were once expected to ease their days when there was no prospect of cure; but as the hospitals expanded their field into research and techniques of surgery and chemotherapy, it became obvious that there were some areas in which they failed. The care of the dying is a case in point; hospice care has evolved to take over an area which the hospital, with its curative ethic, is less able to deal with.

Hospitals today increasingly rehabilitate elderly people and return them to their homes, rather than nurse them bedridden for years. Psychiatric hospitals, once asylums in the literal sense, where mentally ill people were committed to remain for life, now have very few people who are regarded as incurably mentally ill. They, too, have changed their role as places in which people who might be a danger to themselves or to society were effectively imprisoned. Only certain secure units now have this function clearly defined.

The mental handicap hospitals are currently in an emerging phase which will, of necessity, last at least another decade.

Admissions to hospital by virtue of mental handicap alone will no longer be possible, and the Health Service will resist the admissions due to social necessity which have been common in the past. So the community will have to provide respite provisions, for parents and those who give daily care to mentally handicapped children and the more dependent adults, as well as permanent homes. Whether such provision needs to be purpose-built is open to debate. Homeless families are frequently accommodated in private hotels on a temporary basis – often to the open indignation of ratepayers who foot the bills. A place for one mentally handicapped person in times of sudden emergency, sharing, if necessary, with one helper, should not be as difficult as housing a family with four children and often including an expectant mother.

Most areas have small guest houses which could act in this way, and holidays for mentally handicapped people are commonly arranged in accommodation available to all.

Hostels for adults, both young and old, will need to be provided for certain stages in the lives of mentally handicapped people, but in some cases there can be little reason why they should not share facilities already provided by voluntary bodies.

Local authorities do not often, as a matter of course, build hostels in their districts for the ordinary population, although some have done so. Most prefer to consider temporarily homeless single people as transients, catered for by the YMCA, YWCA and Salvation Army, among many other voluntary bodies. The hostel is designed to put a roof over the heads of people, provide food and shelter, on a temporary basis. It should be so regarded for mentally handicapped people, also.

Sheltered Housing

The natural progression from the hostel, in the ordinary course of events, is a move towards a bed-sitting room or flat. Difficult for the many hundreds of working people, it is no less so for mentally handicapped people, but with the essential difference that in any population their numbers are small.

For those with severe disabilities, and those with additional physical handicaps, some special requirements must be made, just as they have traditionally been made for the infirm elderly. Appropriate housing, warmly heated, with manageable access, and with the efficient and unobtrusive supervision of a housekeeper or warden for the full 24 hours if needed, with nursing provided by the community nursing team, would enable many to live outside the hospital. Central catering facilities may or may not be needed, or can be provided for the residents to use as they choose.

This sheltered housing has a defined objective: to provide the dignity of a degree of independence with recognition of the special needs of the residents and, by relieving them of the anxiety of daily problems, leave them free to enjoy their lives as far as their disability allows.

Training Homes

If an amenity for mentally handicapped people is described as a 'training home', it must clearly be training for some objective, usually independent living.

The period may be long or short, as the individual ability of mentally handicapped people of comparable age is more diverse than that of the ordinary person, but once the objective of the training is reached, the need to consolidate by practice is urgent. It is no use setting up a group home training project without previously having acquired the house to which the 'trained' group will go. Far better acquire the house first and devise the training within it.

The training home may well be needed for young people living with parents, to give them additional instruction before they make a move from home which is desired by both parent and child. Their needs will be to accommodate their personal wishes to those of strangers, to learn to get on with other people.

The training units within hospitals or attached to them will, in the natural course of events, become less necessary for mentally handicapped people of moderate ability, because they will not have been admitted there in the first instance. Hospital training units currently prepare people who have suffered a mental illness for re-entry into society, and they could provide the services required for people who become mentally handicapped as a result of accident or infection.

It may be that new techniques will be discovered which will enable even those long resident in mental handicap hospitals, with intractable behaviour problems or with conditions at present considered unamenable to any known medical or psychological treatment, to receive some individual training and to move out into the community, but the total numbers of these people will become less year by year as the community fulfils its obligations.

Foster Homes
Very seriously mentally handicapped infants receive the same intensive care as others. I do not propose to enter the debate upon this 'same care'. Society does not yet have a commonly accepted view regarding the advisability of survival of grievously afflicted infants, nor upon the parental and professional role in this dilemma. What is clear is that if the infant survives with a mental handicap of great severity, there is no logical medical reason why he should be segregated at that time or later in his life, from the infant who survives with a physical disability, by being despatched to a special mental handicap unit.

Like the blind child or the deaf child, he will need special facilities, but he does not need, nor should he be condemned to, a life spent only among those similarly afflicted. He needs, first, a roof over his head and a place to live. All else can be added later. With the acceptance of the disability of mental handicap, we have seen an increasing number of families prepared to offer foster homes to children who, for one reason or another, are not able to be cared for by their natural parents. These fostering parents find satisfaction and fulfilment in providing care for a child with special needs. Their parenting role requires support services from all professionals: medical, nursing and social services at all times, and education services in the school years and in early adult life. The need for a home for that child when he is fully adult must also be planned for.

2 The Need for Numerical Planning

When considering the future of homes in the community designed to give a reasonable expectation of life-long residence, what numbers of people must we cater for? If we assume the incidence of children born mentally handicapped to be about 3 per 1,000 with severe handicap and the identification of mental handicap at school-leaving age to be 10 per 1,000 of all degrees of handicap, both mild and severe, we can anticipate that the present known population of mentally handicapped people will increase each year by new births which are not balanced by deaths. Short of a common policy regarding the application of the results of genetic and biological research, there is no reason to expect a change in the foreseeable future, and the mentally handicapped will enjoy a greater expectation of long life in common with the rest of us.

In February 1981, Hansard quoted in the 12th to 15th January 1981 reports a reply by Sir George Young on the cost of mental handicap expenditure for the year 1978–79. In hospitals (on both in- and out-patient services) the cost was £227.1 millions (a 3.8 percentage of all NHS expenditure), and on the residential service provisions of the Social Services it was £32.9 millions.

As the population of mental handicap hospitals falls, and more effective use is made of the remaining revenue expenditure, those figures could be reversed, especially if, in the next century, the remaining severely afflicted and elderly mentally handicapped people receive care in medical units designed for the ordinary population.

Planning for future needs is based upon past experience and predictions from statistical data. The difficulty is that there are few accurate figures upon which to base forward plans. We can assume an incidence from reliable research of a percentage of all births, but we cannot know the extent to which environmental and educational factors will render those born handicapped more or less so, nor predict accurately what their continuing needs will be.

Only broad outlines are available, as is made apparent by the Office of Health Economics, a private body set up by the British Pharmaceutical Industry, in their report, *Mental Handicap – Ways Forward*, 1978. For the whole population of the United Kingdom the number of mentally handicapped people they estimate is 'probably 400,000', based upon those 'who have at some stage in their lives come to the notice of providing authorities as being handicapped or educationally subnormal'.

They say that on the assumption of percentage incidence, the full number of people with some degree of mental handicap is likely to be approximately one million people, but that many of these function sufficiently well to live independently.

Assuming that most of this group of people live at home with their families and that the older members of this group have never appeared in any statistical records, the need for somewhere to live when parents are no longer able to provide a home can be seen as a major planning problem for the future.

In the study quoted, the Office of Health Economics base their predictions upon the statements and figures for services existing in 1969 in England and Wales, where the *actual* number of children attending special educational schools and Junior Training Centres is given as 23,400, plus an *estimated* 500 infants under five years receiving day care – approximately 24,000 in all. Adults – that is people who had left school in 1969 and were living in the community and attending Adult Training Centres – numbered 24,500.

The suggested increase in places for education and adult occupation centres up to the end of the century is estimated to be increased up to 3,900 places for infants under five in day care or education, 27,400 in general special education, and 63,700 places for adults who have left school.

There are additional figures for those expected to be in hospital care in the future, and it is the inclusion of an estimated hospital population of school-age children of 2,900 which illustrates the difficulty surrounding statistical predictions. Since the study was published it has been decreed that *no* child will be admitted to hospital by virtue of mental handicap alone.

Nevertheless, even such approximate guidance reveals a very great number of mentally handicapped people who are expected to live in the community.

Already the situation in Adult Centres of all kinds presents acute problems. Without any criteria for discharge from such a centre, except open or sheltered employment, the waiting lists grow longer and longer, and young adults living at home and unable to find places are denied any structured courses of education or training.

3 Providing the Funds

Government forward financial planning has included an element from the Government Joint Finance Funds. *Care in the Community* quotes the allocation as £68.5 millions in 1981–82 and £71.0 millions in 1982–83, of which one-third is to be devoted to mental handicap.

The purpose of Joint Finance funding is to enable the transfer of some part of patient care from the hospital or other NHS services to local authorities, or to voluntary bodies which are sponsored by local authorities. Joint Finance funds the capital costs of projects and the subsequent running costs for two years afterwards, but the fundamental principle is that the continued financial responsibility will then be accepted by the local authority or by the voluntary organisation. It is this forward commitment which has made some authorities and voluntary bodies chary of initiating new projects, although others have 'boldly gone where none have gone before'.

Joint Finance funds are not normally extended to provide local authority housing, but it may be considered for schemes which remove people from hospital care into the responsibility of Social Services Departments, and this possibility is being exploited. At the moment Social Services Departments in many areas are exploring methods of removing patients who could return to their home area if suitable places were available. If such transfers were accompanied by a transfer of funds some of the difficulties would disappear, although already others are taking their place. Hospital staff, greatly depleted and left with an increasing number of highly dependent older people and severely disturbed younger adults, cannot see how the time and resources needed to prepare this category of hospital residents can be found amid the pressures of daily care and supervision of other patients. Such preparation may take years on a one to one basis.

Some medical and nursing staff openly question whether the social services staff – much more mobile and non-resident in comparison with the hospital staff – even if supported by the community nursing expertise of mental handicap district teams, can cope with people with severe mental handicap which is sometimes complicated by superimposed medical conditions, such as epilepsy or diabetes. They fear that years of patient training, followed by a failure in community living and a return to the hospital, will further disrupt any security of the groups left in hospital care.

The Social Services Departments, acknowledging the sound preparation given in hospitals before discharge, are growing more confident as they gain experience and log up a catalogue of success; they wish to be given greater opportunity to provide for mentally handicapped people from hospitals. At the same time, local authorities are being urged not to forget the continuing needs of those currently resident with their parents. There is still a disparity in the financial position of parents who undertake years of care of their own child, even if they receive all the available state benefits appropriate, and the financial support available to those who undertake the care of children in need either as foster parents or in hospital.

Salaried hospital staff are not expected to give 24-hour service, 7 days a week, 365 days per year; their salaries are based upon a working week of under forty hours. Foster parents, responsible for care on a 24-hour basis, are paid a sufficiently generous allowance, in addition to the statutory benefits for the child, to pay for modest domestic help, and are spared financial anxiety, rightly so, though some notable abuses by individuals of the financial rewards have come to light.

It is obviously unjust that whilst a child received into a hospital is no longer a financial charge upon his parents, even though the cost of his care may be very high, the child who is severely handicapped living at home with his own parents is less well provided for.

Local authorities are today inheriting past patterns. After 1971 they began to implement their responsibilities by building hostels which required resident staff, and often needed a high ratio of staff to residents. As these were quite large amenities, and often purpose-built, they were sometimes sited where land was more available, on the outskirts of towns and not in the central position of ordinary council houses. They have quickly become 'Homes' with a capital letter.

With prospects of joint funds becoming available and the experience they have gained, many Social Services Departments are now faced with the dilemma of how to keep faith with their own ratepayers in providing the best value for money spent, how to meet the wishes of parents in the area with children at home and older family members in nearby hospitals, or in some cases, very remote hospitals, and how to meet the challenges faced by the employment of staff. The hospital is training community nurses, still hospital based and salaried; district nurses and health visitors may be attached to the general practitioners' districts; adult education services, with participation in training centres, have instructors and teachers responsible to the Education Authority. The number of social work staff concerned is being reduced by financial demands, and the demands of administration increasingly force the social work load upon relatively untrained and part-time helpers to give actual personal help to those they serve.

Some use this situation to urge both the formation of a central administrative body, a Ministry of Mental Handicap, as an overall co-ordinating force, and an increase of social service staff.

From what I have seen and studied, the major common factor in successful schemes has been the *local* liaison and local knowledge and experience. In many cases the initiatives have come from the parents who have used the democratic rights of the citizen to make local authorities aware of their needs. The most successful, however, have not stopped there. They have gone ahead with self-help projects, with varying success, but with the supreme merit of enterprise and originality which contributes so greatly to knowledge and provides a model, good or bad, to be followed or avoided by others. The concept of another bureaucratic machine to make the whole service more efficient is laudable, but nothing in past experience has shown that any government machinery is conducive to lively and original thinking; if it occurs at all, it will be so modified, investigated by committees and ponderously planned, that it either dies at birth or emerges after so prolonged a gestation that it has all the problems of being out of date before it sees the light of day.

There are many successful small projects fulfilling local needs. They are unresearched and unrecorded in most cases, and must attribute some of their success to this very fact. If a project is commenced as a research project, and funded on that basis, it is right and proper that it should be correctly recorded and the results published to justify the often not inconsiderable expenditure involved. The past ten years have seen many such projects with recorded results.

We cannot afford, however, to go on collecting data. What we need for the future is to take hold of the local problem, select and apply what is relevant from the experience of others, define what is needed, seek out what aid is available and get on with the job. If it succeeds, it can be repeated there in the area for which it was designed. Missionary zeal to impose a local pattern nationwide should be resisted by both the originators and local planners. Nor should Government aid the analysis of the increasing number of projects by additional allocations to research workers and staff. We already have a vast amount of data, and more statistics and research findings are not likely to produce a single extra 'home of their own' for mentally handicapped people. Detached analysis of statistics may provide some ideas for proper use of funds, but the provision of a real home will rest as it has always done, with the people on the spot.

4 Providing the Support

The earlier pages of this book have been devoted to accounts of the preparation for independent living and have demonstrated what can be achieved in a comparatively short period of time to equip mentally handicapped people to live in homes of their own. Few of those participating in training schemes needed longer than two years to acquire skills previously denied them, even after many years of hospital life.

In some cases, after properly designed courses of training, a period as short as three months has been sufficient to allow a long-stay resident from a mental handicap hospital to take a tenancy in a council-provided house, sharing with other mentally handicapped people.

These groups should be small – four seems to be the ideal number – and self-selected, so that they live with friends of their own choice, thus minimising the friction of incompatible personalities. Under these conditions the skills acquired by those who have lived together are quickly passed on to a new resident joining the group at a later date.

Mentally handicapped people are often intuitive about each other, anticipating needs and supplying them without reference to other helpers. In some cases they are the best teachers. This is particularly the case when behaviour difficulties arise. In several instances I was able to observe how a resident exhibiting mildly noisy or extravagant behaviour was quietly checked by one of her friends; younger women, in general, are more likely to 'act up' to attract attention, and their friends are quick to protect them from the consequences of this unacceptable behaviour.

Most studies of accommodation for mentally handicapped people have, of necessity, been confined to the larger units which prepare people for independent living. Once they move out into the community, mentally handicapped people are tenants of ordinary houses, entitled to privacy and respect as individuals. Nevertheless it is impossible to assess the success, or otherwise, of the preparation, without seeing for oneself how well the residents manage to cope. I am extremely conscious of the privilege accorded to me by those who invited me into their homes, and grateful to them for their hospitality. Their names and the location of their homes have been suppressed for this reason.

No community provision can succeed without the support services required, no matter how excellent the preparation and training of residents and the careful planning of the houses.

As early as 1968, in their report on residential care, the Directors of the National Association for Retarded Children, New York, stated:

> Responsibility for the care of persons who have returned to the community should not be relinquished by the residential facility until assistance is assured from some other source.
>
> The community placement should guarantee at least as much, if not more, in the way of services and programmes as the residential facility from which the individual came.

The years of dependence upon others, and the system which produces an apathetic acceptance of a routine, are only overcome by continuous and rigorous training. Reversion to the earlier state can occur very rapidly if the individual is not given adequate support and unless the group of which he is a member is carefully selected; the 'key' supporting person must have genuine and continuing interest in his welfare if independence is to be successfully achieved.

It is just this fear, of a gradual deterioration, due to staff changes or to a slackening of the original enthusiasm, which leads many parents to choose *any* form of residence which appears to offer continuity and therefore familiarity to their mentally handicapped family members, of any age.

Writing in the newspaper of the North West Region of the Royal Society for Mentally Handicapped Children and Adults, in October 1980, one parent explains why he and his wife arranged for their daughter aged 27, to leave them to live in a house run by the Home Farm Trust, With the example before them of a relative, suddenly taken into a subnormality hospital at an advanced age on the death of her surviving parent, and the consequent suffering and distress in which she ended her life, this young woman's parents have prepared her, during the past years, for a life apart from them. They have decided upon an establishment which will offer continuous supervision within a closed community, rather than an ordinary house run by the occupants with support from local authority services.

I have been fortunate to see some projects with excellent support systems, but we all know that these are not universal, and that even the best are precariously at risk by reason of economic and other factors. Mentally handicapped people are essentially vulnerable members of any community.

If we are to make provision for them to live among us, the commitment to do so must be absolute, the resolution to continue to give the help and support their changing needs require must be constant, and the controlling administration firm and farseeing.

As the NARC Report, New York, (previously quoted) reminds us, 'The process of dehumanisation can occur in a community facility as well as in residential facilities. Too often, in an attempt to place an individual in a community setting, the safeguards necessary to ensure that the needs of the mentally retarded person are in fact met have not always been established.' It is in the establishment of these safeguards that the success or failure of the whole system of community residence of mentally handicapped people will be judged.

Cooperation is the key to this aspect. Community mental handicap teams, local voluntary services, local authority amenities of all kinds, education, leisure, transport, the nationalised industries supplying services, and commercial enterprises, all contribute to the quality of life of every citizen. The mentally handicapped residents among us will be affected equally by these various services.

We must ensure that they have access to whatever exists for the rest of the community. To do so often means the appointment of one or more salaried co-ordinators who are aware of what is available, can identify gaps in the services and plan how they may be filled.

The co-ordinators will need not only a comprehensive grasp of local conditions and statutory benefits, but an intimate knowledge of the individuals who need help. They will also need to have respect for personal qualities and differences and be prepared to accept their client's choice of life style. Independence is as precious to mentally handicapped people as to others, and, however limited in degree by their ability, must be accorded in full.

That this is possible is amply demonstrated by the many small family homes described in this book; from the bungalow in which Joey and Ernie – both grievously physically afflicted in addition to their mental handicap – were enabled to live like other people, with their daily family care provided for by their friends who shared their home with the support of a key helper, to the men and women I met who were living quite independently in single person flats.

All had needed patient preparation, special education programmes designed to develop their individual abilities, encouragement and approval to maintain their hardly acquired confidence after long years of total dependence. Their example is a shining proof that life outside the walls of the hospital is the right of all mentally handicapped people who do not require more medical care than the rest of us – and also for some who do, provided that we genuinely care enough to make it possible.

5 The Factors for Success

The original inspiration for this book was simply the interest and excitement I experienced on my visits to two ventures described in detail in the earlier part of this book: the bungalow home of Joey Deacon and his friends, and the preparation for community life of the young people at Pengwern Hall.

I saw these projects from the outside, as an informed observer, and was admitted as a friend by those concerned because of previous acquaintance. In recording the real situation in the home life of a family one must be able to feel at ease, to be accepted to a degree which enables the family to express their feelings and to behave naturally, as they would to any other familiar visitor.

It is not enough to study the reports and records of new enterprises, nor can the success or failure be estimated by an analysis of results. Both successes and failures turn upon so many factors intrinsic in each situation which may not be repeatable elsewhere.

As the work of recording the two ventures at St. Lawrence's and Pengwern Hall proceeded, I became aware that I was attempting to isolate the ingredients for success which might be repeated in other communities.

When I extended my studies into other areas – for example, into the council houses in which mentally handicapped people were living – I began to see that there are very few common factors for success. Enormous variations in local conditions, in the abilities of residents and in emotional responses, make it impossible to lay down absolute standards. Nevertheless I am personally convinced of certain essentials, if mentally handicapped people are to live in reasonable contentment and happiness outside an institution.

We need first of all to consider what they themselves would choose as their place of residence, and be aware that this choice will depend upon their personal needs at any point in their lives.

Childhood

Young children need the loving security of a stable environment which is sufficiently familiar to be taken for granted, so that the energy for learning and exploration is freed from daily uncertainties. The child needs to know that whatever adventures the day may hold for him, his bed awaits him in his usual room, a familiar face will greet him when he wakes and his days are in some measure predictable.

For mentally handicapped children this quiet routine gives pattern and shape to the days and a framework within which the special activities designed to develop and educate can best be carried out.

In the early days of childhood, stability is probably best achieved in the family environment, and if the natural parents are not able to care for the child, a foster family may be the best, no matter how severe the handicap. As the child grows, the need to widen the field of experience becomes greater, and by puberty, the young adult begins to challenge the accepted family pattern and to need an increasing degree of independence. He also needs, and prefers, the company of those of similar age to himself.

Adolescence

Adolescence gives the second chance to change the attitudes of childhood and to learn new skills. For these and other reasons, it may be the time for a move into a hostel situation, perhaps for the weekdays only at first, returning home at weekends, or perhaps for spending a night or two away from the environment of childhood. Ordinary young adults are prone to sudden departures from home at this time, and if unprepared suffer accordingly.

Mentally handicapped young people need a degree of help to adjust to the demands of modern life, and some residential units with staff will be needed at this time. These hostel units should not be large, and should not be designed to provide a permanent home. They may perhaps incorporate self-contained flats, and even accommodation for married couples, should some of the mentally handicapped residents subsequently marry, but the very fact of the increased size of the buildings required, and their association with a changing intake of people for training and education, precludes them from classification as ordinary family homes.

They can, however, prove an essential temporary home for emergencies, serving the same function as a small guest house, to which people can repair when some unplanned emergency arises, and where they can await more permanent arrangements.

Adulthood

The time is long past when purpose built units for mentally handicapped people should be considered. Every local housing authority already supplies, to a greater or lesser extent, housing for people with special needs, such as the elderly, and adapts ordinary housing for handicapped people, such as those who are blind or physically disabled. Mentally handicapped people require neither more nor less than this degree of concern.

Equally, the very large majority do not need to have staff resident with them. Few people today regard resident staff as a necessary component of a normal family home. Smaller, more convenient homes have rendered domestic staff unnecessary, except in unusual circumstances, or at times of special crises in family life; help is provided as matter of course by local authorities for their tenants with special needs: a warden in charge of a number of units for elderly people, for example, or social-work support for those in more immediate need.

Once living in the community, nothing more than this type of neighbourly help is needed by mentally handicapped people, provided their preparation has been well and thoroughly carried out and some concerned observation of their changing needs at different ages in life is maintained.

There is at present a divergence of opinion as to whether support should be provided by volunteer helpers, by professionally trained social services staff, or by other neighbourhood services such as the community nursing staff.

There are arguments in favour of all or none of these, and some may be dictated by expediency. At a time of financial restraint the prevailing decision may be to choose what appears to be the least costly. The first essential is to decide what is best, and what is best is what is most fitted for a particular purpose at a particular time.

In providing a home for a particular person, or group of people, we need to decide what is best for them with regard to what they themselves see as best for them. No easy task as, unconsciously, we may be deciding what would be best for ourselves in their situation, instead of what they would see as best.

They need a reasonable standard of comfort and the design of a house which enables this to be achieved without sophisticated equipment or technical knowledge. They need privacy and security for the personal possessions which they value. They may need the companionship of others to a greater or lesser extent, and independence of action again in line with what they feel to be in accordance with their abilities.

Some will find decision-making stressful even in small things, and will be unable to deal with this. In most cases these less independent spirits find another resident who likes to make the daily routine decisions and is happy to do so. It may be a mistake for the outside observer or support professional to attempt to confer more independence on one who does not want it.

The best we can provide will give the greatest possible degree of contentment in living, and if we have truly considered what is the best provision, we can then turn our minds to obtaining it from what already exists and obtaining the best value for the cost involved.

I am convinced that we do not need specially designed homes for most of the mentally handicapped people who live among us. They do not need a specialist medical and nursing, dental or chiropody service; they merely need made available to them the services which already exist. The school dental service, for example, could usefully be extended for them.

The ability of most mentally handicapped people today, particularly those who have received full time appropriate education since the 1970 Handicapped Pupils Education Act provided for them, is far in advance of those born earlier and who were denied the chance of any individual help to enable them to learn and improve upon the disabling effect of their handicap.

The solution in the past to the ultimate residential needs of mentally handicapped people has been to tidy them away out of sight, a consequence of the social policies which incarcerated the indigent and senile into the Poor Law institution. Some, alas, will now never emerge from the hospital care which was provided for them with the best intentions and which, for many, did indeed give them a better chance for mere survival. Sometimes, too, it brought a degree of happiness which would not have been possible outside in the poverty of the years of depression which have followed two world wars. Now, however, with increasing knowledge of methods of education and of the environmental factors which influence handicap, a better way of caring has been emerging.

Those now in the education system, and the young adults emerging at sixteen or nineteen years of age, are less likely than the rest of us to leave the parental home through the natural process of marriage and a family of their own. We have to recognise this and work to fulfil the obligation of their life-time needs for independence which as a civilised society we have undertaken on their behalf.

It is by no means a one-sided bargain. The need to overcome the obstacles presented by carrying the burdens of the less able stimulates original solutions and often widens the horizons of knowledge as an incidental which benefits the non-handicapped and handicapped able.

'The proper study of mankind is Man,' and men and women of all degrees of ability are equally subject to the duties and responsibilities of humanity, sharing equally in the right to a *chance* of a good life. Not all will achieve it, but all should be given the opportunity to make what they can of their lives.

APPENDICES

Statistics

Reference has been made throughout this book to the estimated number of mentally handicapped people for whom forward planning of provisions for education, training, support and residence will be needed. There are very considerable difficulties in obtaining accurate data for many reasons.

The only reliable figures are those for children now receiving special education by virtue of mental handicap. Before 1970, only those with an intelligence quotient of over 50 would have featured in these figures, and only those between the statutory ages of admission and discharge from state education. Severely handicapped children of school age were eligible for entry to Junior Training Centres, and upon reaching school leaving age, to Adult Training Centres, but there was no *compulsion* to attend either; many parents made alternative arrangements for severely retarded children, and many severely retarded adults did not choose to attend Training Centres.

The figures for children and adults in mental handicap hospitals reflect a changing population. At any time there will be some who are admitted on a temporary basis, to help at a time of family crisis, or to give a short respite to families. The data for 'adults and children' is also subject to change, as once the child attains sixteen years of age his occupancy is transferred to the adult figures. This fact alone has accounted for a high percentage drop in numbers of children in mental handicap hospitals in the past ten years. They are still there, but no longer counted as children.

The definition of mental handicap is very wide and covers many conditions, none of which at the present time is subject to mandatory notification. Some local authorities have been compiling registers of those who have come to the notice of their

Social Services Departments as needing services, but for forward planning, local authorities need to rely on their special education figures.

Again, the needs of mentally handicapped people are as diverse as the rest of the population and change materially throughout their lives. It may not even be accurate to base future needs upon past experience. Large residential units in the past may actually have *produced* the highly dependent people for whom hospital accommodation is needed, and the smaller community units, designed to remove people from hospital, may, by encouraging independence, preclude the need for such admissions in the future. The tables of incidence in the normal population of 3 to 4 per thousand mentally handicapped people provide little guidance on the type of service needed, apart from special education from the earliest years.

Future requirements will be modified by the success of education and training, by improved environmental conditions, and by wider application of genetic and biochemical research.

Government reports and special committees present selected statistical data in the relevant field of their studies, and details of some of these are given in the Bibliography.

For those who wish to use statistical data which have been reliably collected, it is essential to frame the question needing an answer. If the question is too general there may not be an answer. For example, if one asks how many mentally handicapped babies have been born this year, the reply will of necessity be on the lines of the expected incidence and may be inaccurate. If one asks how many children have been identified as *needing* special education by virtue of mental handicap this year, the answer will be more accurate.

Again, the recording procedure means that all *published* statistics are considerably delayed and not usually available until some months *after* the end of the period in question.

However, for those who wish to pursue the study of the elusive statistical data, the source for national figures is the Government Statistical Service, Central Statistical Office, Great George Street, London SW1. To obtain *any* answer, it is necessary accurately to define and refine the question, so that the appropriate department has the opportunity of providing an answer. The situation locally is similar. A thorough study of the situation is needed before deciding what question to ask, but there may not always be an accessible answer.

For example, if the Housing Department is asked how many mentally handicapped people live in council houses, they will have no idea; there is no analysis of ordinary council residents by medical or other categories, and several families in council houses may have mentally handicapped people living at home for whom no special services have ever been requested. If the question is, 'How many people have been allocated council houses because they are mentally handicapped?' the answer may well be known, but it may not be given to the casual enquirer, either from a wish to preserve the privacy of the tenants, or for the protection of a housing project for mentally handicapped people which is still in an early, vulnerable phase.

Not all statistics are 'damn' lies', but all are subject to many interpretations, and it is for this reason that so many figures quoted for all areas of mental handicap often appear contradictory. The most commonly quoted sources of statistical data are given below:

Government Statistical Service
The United Kingdom in Figures. 1981 Edition. Central Office of Information 1981. HMSO.

Parliamentary Questions
November 16th 1981. Written reply to Robert Kilroy-Silk (Ormskirk). The number of people in mental handicap hospitals for the years 1976–1980.

Mental Handicap – Ways Forward. 1978.
Prevalence tables, rates of mental handicap. (Page 9, Table 2.) Office of Health Economics.

Mental Handicap: Progress, Problems and Priorities. DHSS 1980.
Estimated numbers given as 'just over three per thousand' needing services, '15,000 hospital residents able to live outside with appropriate support . . . about 5,000 severely handicapped adults living at home.'

Bibliography

Books

BARANYAY, EILEEN. *Fifty Years of Harperbury Hospital*, 1981, Royal Society for Mentally Handicapped Children and Adults.

BARANYAY, EILEEN. *The Mentally Handicapped Adolescent: The Slough Project*, 1971, Pergamon Press.

BARANYAY, EILEEN. *Towards a Full Life. Report of a Survey*, 1981, Royal Society for Mentally Handicapped Children and Adults.

BOARD OF DIRECTORS of the National Association for Retarded Children. *Policy Statements on Residential Care*, October 1968, 420, Lexington Avenue, New York 10017.

DEACON, JOSEPH. *Tongue Tied*, 1974, Royal Society for Mentally Handicapped Children and Adults.

DEPARTMENT OF HEALTH AND SOCIAL SECURITY. *Better Services for the Mentally Handicapped*, 1971, CMND 4683, HMSO.

DEPARTMENT OF HEALTH AND SOCIAL SECURITY. *Care in the Community. A Consultative Document*, July 1981, HMSO.

FELCE, D., SMITH, J., & KUSHLICK, A. *The Evaluation of the Wessex Experiment*, Beacon, Autumn 1981, Home Counties North Region, Royal Society for Mentally Handicapped Children and Adults.

GATHERCOLE, C. E. *Group Homes, Staffed and Unstaffed*, 1981, British Institute of Mental Handicap.

GATHERCOLE, C. E. *Leisure, Social Integration and Volunteers*, 1981, British Institute for Mental Handicap.

HEGINBOTHAM, C. *Housing for Mentally Handicapped People*, 1980, Royal Society for Mentally Handicapped Children and Adults.

HEGINBOTHAM, C. *Housing Projects for Mentally Handicapped People*, 1981, Centre on Environment for the Handicapped, 126 Albert Street, London NW1 7NI.

HIGH WYCOMBE SOCIETY for Mentally Handicapped Children and Adults. *Survey of the Needs of the Mentally Handicapped Resident in Wycombe District*, 1980.

INSKIP, HAMPDEN. *Family Support Services for Physically and Mentally Handicapped People in their Own Homes*, 1981, Leonard Cheshire Foundation, Bedford Square Press.

MITTLER, PETER. *Mental Handicap: Progress, Problems and Priorities*, December 1980, DHSS, Room C414, Alexander Fleming House, Elephant and Castle, London SE1 6BY.

NATIONAL FEDERATION OF HOUSING ASSOCIATIONS. *Guide to Housing Associations*, 30 Southampton Street, London WC2.

NEAL, H. *New Era Housing Association*, Beacon, Spring 1980, Home Counties North Region, Royal Society for Mentally Handicapped Children and Adults.

NORTHUMBERLAND AREA HEALTH AUTHORITY. *NHS Residential Accommodation for Mentally Handicapped People*, April 1981, East Cottingwood, Morpeth, Northumberland, NE61 2PD.

OFFICE OF HEALTH ECONOMICS. *Mental Hendicap – Ways Forward*, 1978, 162 Regent Street, London W1.

PEARLMAN, DELLA. *No Choice: Library Services for the Mentally Handicapped*, 1981, The Library Association.

RACE, D. G. & D. M. *The Cherries Group Home*, 1979, HMSO.

ROYAL SOCIETY FOR MENTALLY HANDICAPPED CHILDREN AND ADULTS. *The Mencap Homes Foundation*, 1982.

REPORT OF A WORKING PARTY. *Working Together. Partnerships in Local Social Services*, 1981, Bedford Square Press.

SCOTT, CAROL. *Work Experience for Mentally Handicapped People*, 1982, Royal Society for Mentally Handicapped Children and Adults.

SCOTTISH SOCIETY FOR THE MENTALLY HANDICAPPED. *Annual Report 1979–80*, 13, Elmbank Street, Glasgow G2 4QA.

SHENNAN, VICTORIA (Ed.). *Directory of Residential Accommodation for Mentally Handicapped People in England,*

Wales and Northern Ireland, 1982, Royal Society For Mentally Handicapped Children and Adults.

SHENNAN, VICTORIA. *Mental Handicap Nursing and Care*, 1980, Souvenir Press.

SIMON, G. B. (Ed.). *Local Services for Mentally Handicapped People*, 1981, British Institute of Mental Handicap, Wolverhampton Road, Kidderminster, Worcs.

SOUTH EAST REGION, Royal Society for Mentally Handicapped Children and Adults. *Home Sweet Home?*, November 1980, 34 Surrey Street, Croydon CR0 1RJ.

WEINBERG, MARTIN. *Pengwern Hall*, 1982, Royal Society for Mentally Handicapped Children and Adults.

WHEELER, RENEE (Ed.). *Planning for the Future. Survey of the London Borough of Barnet*, 1976, Royal Society for Mentally Handicapped Children and Adults.

WHELAN, EDWARD, & SPEAKE, BARBARA. *Getting to Work*, 1981, Souvenir Press.

WHELAN, EDWARD, & SPEAKE, BARBARA. *Learning to Cope*, 1979, Souvenir Press.

WILLIAMS, PAUL, & SHOULTZ, BONNIE. *We Can Speak for Ourselves: Self-Advocacy by Mentally Handicapped People*, 1982, Souvenir Press.

Reports and Articles

Improving the Quality of Services for Mentally Handicapped People – a Checklist of Standards, 1980, DHSS.

NATIONAL DEVELOPMENT GROUP (1978). *Helping Mentally Handicapped People in Hospital*, 1978, HMSO.

FELCE, D., KUSHLICK, A. & SMITH, J. 'Planning and evaluation of a programme of community based residences for severely mentally handicapped people'. Health Care Evaluation Research Team, Wessex Regional Health Authority.

Report of the Committee of Enquiry into Mental Handicap Nursing and Care (The Jay Report), 1979, CMND 7468, HMSO.

MATHIESON, J. S. & BLUNDEN, R. 'Nimrod, piloting a course towards a community life', *Health and Social Services Journal*, January 25th 1980, pp. 122–124.

Mental Handicap in Wales. Applied Research Unit, Annual Report 1980/81 (The Nimrod Service), The White House, 44, Cowbridge Road East, Cardiff CF1 9DU.

WELSH OFFICE. *Report of a Joint Working Party on the provision of a Community Based Mental Handicap Service in South Glamorgan,* Cardiff. Welsh Office 1978.

Development of Health Service Residential and Day Care Facilities for Mentally Handicapped People. Winchester and Central Hampshire Health District.

Film and Video

NORTHUMBERLAND AREA HEALTH AUTHORITY. Tape slide programme and video presentation available on the Ashington project, housing children in the community. From: AHA Headquarters, East Cottingwood, Morpeth.